SWIM
Wild & Free

BLOOMSBURY SPORT
Bloomsbury Publishing Plc
50 Bedford Square, London, WC1B 3DP, UK
29 Earlsfort Terrace, Dublin 2, Ireland

BLOOMSBURY, BLOOMSBURY SPORT and the
Diana logo are trademarks of Bloomsbury Publishing Plc

This edition published 2022

A catalogue record for this book is available from the
British Library

Library of Congress Cataloguing-in-Publication data has
been applied for

ISBN: 9781-3994-0040-4 eBook: 978-1-3994-0039-8

2 4 6 8 10 9 7 5 3 1

Typeset in Spectral by Luke Griffin
Printed and bound in China by Toppan Leefung Printing Co

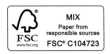

To find out more about our authors and books visit
www.bloomsbury.com and sign up for our newsletters

SWIM
Wild & Free

A Practical Guide to
Swimming Outdoors
365 Days a Year

SIMON GRIFFITHS

BLOOMSBURY SPORT
LONDON · OXFORD · NEW YORK · NEW DELHI · SYDNEY

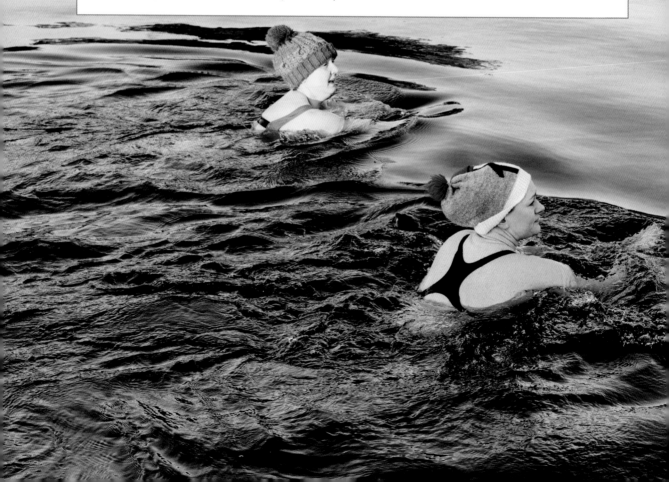

CONTENTS

FOREWORD

Nature blesses us by providing both the most beautiful scenes and many ways to interact with them. Outdoor swimming is perhaps the best of these. As an open water swimmer, I competed for Great Britain at the Tokyo 2020 Olympic Games as well as in numerous other international competitions. Open water swimming has always pushed me out of my comfort zone in a terrifying way, but also one that allows me to show myself what I am truly made of. For me, swimming in nature brings peace and serenity, but also a thrill of excitement. Getting to share those feelings with other people only adds to the experience.

This book provides all you need to explore the ins and outs of outdoor swimming. Whether you are a complete beginner looking to take that first dip or a seasoned swimmer hoping to get some tips for everything from a mile swim to the Channel crossing, this book will take you through it all. Simon Griffiths has a wealth of outdoor swimming knowledge, all of which is now in your hands...

So get ready, and get your wetsuit or your costume out. Have the thermos flask and cake on standby and brace yourself for the fantastic world that is outdoor swimming.

ALICE DEARING

Olympic marathon swimmer, World Junior Open Water Champion (2016), co-founder of the Black Swimming Association (BSA) and first black woman to represent Team GB in swimming at an Olympic Games.

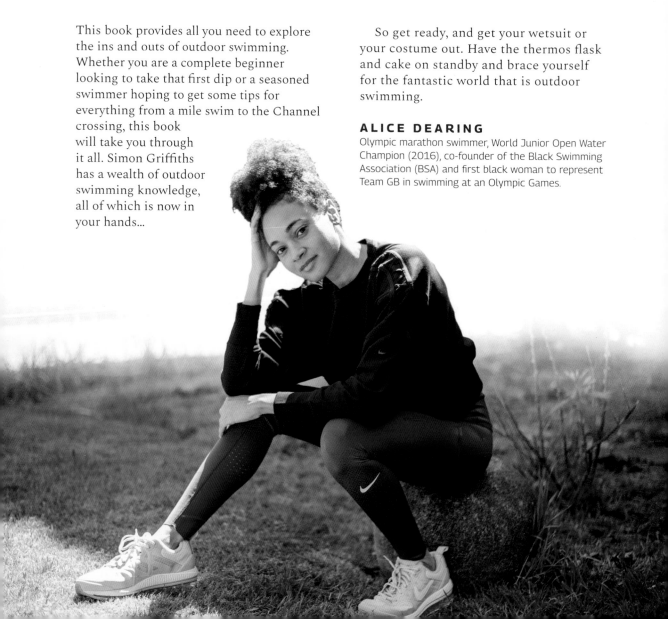

WELCOME

Hello and welcome to the wonderful world of outdoor swimming. From head-up breaststroker and frog's-eye observer of nature to high-speed, head-down competitive freestyler, outdoor swimming is a fabulous, inclusive activity for all ages and all types of swimmer, and there is space in the open water for everyone. When you combine swimming with immersion in natural water you set yourself up for a lifetime of magical experiences. Whether you are dipping your toe in the water for the first time or have already taken the plunge and are wondering what other outdoor swimming adventures await you, this book will show you how.

As you progress, you will learn how to adapt to swimming in cooler water (see Chapter 6) and how to cope with the challenges you might meet when swimming wild and free. For the more advanced, we've included details of how to design your own training programme to help you swim faster and further. While swimming is beautifully simple and natural, there is a lifetime of learning and exploration ahead of you.

You have probably heard that swimming in cold water is good for you, that it boosts your mood and may even help protect you against dementia. We look at the science behind these claims and share the stories of people whose lives have been transformed by outdoor swimming.

Imagine a caged bird that escapes: the sense of freedom, the ability to fly anywhere, new views and opportunities for adventure. At the same time, it faces new dangers. It must learn to watch out for predators and adapt to changing weather conditions. Escaping the pool and becoming an outdoor swimmer is something like this. No longer bounded by tiled walls and cocooned in tepid, chemically disinfected water, you're free to explore the 70 per cent of the planet that's covered by water. It's how we've swum for thousands of years. Pools are a recent invention. Expect glorious sunrises from the water, mental and physical rejuvenation from embracing the cold and exciting challenges. Revel in your freedom, but take responsibility for your safety.

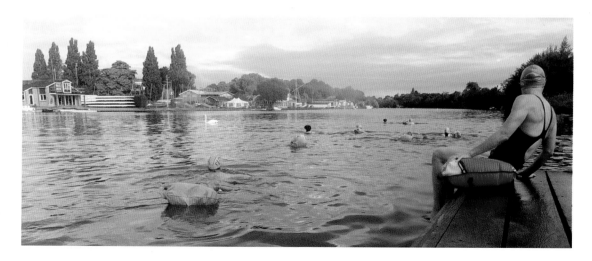

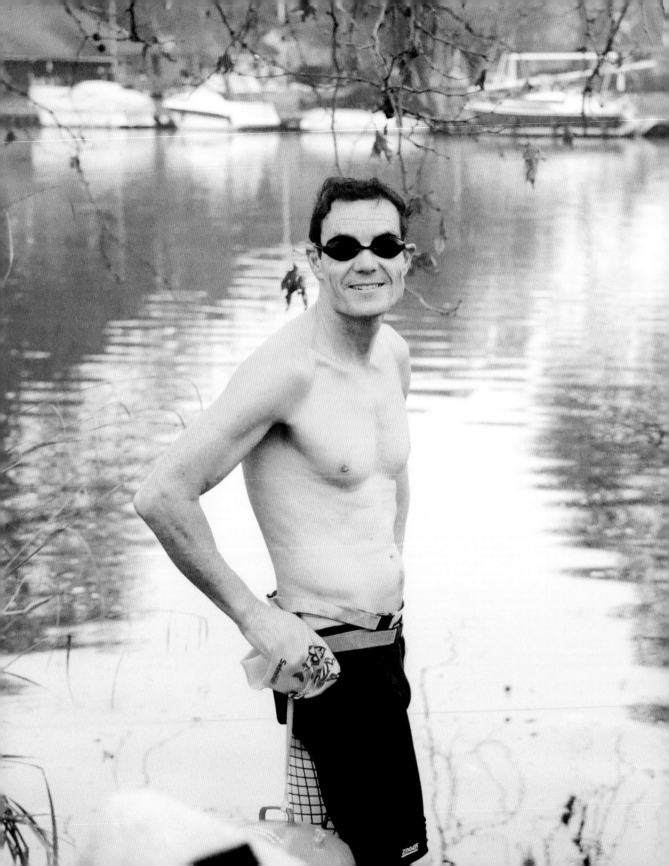

A LIFELONG PASSION FOR SWIMMING

I've always swum. When I'm near water, I feel compelled to get in and swim. I love the way I can move in water. It's comforting, relaxing and restorative. I struggle with gyms. The thought of heaving lumps of iron around fills me with dread. But put me in the water and I can happily swim for hours. I'm grateful and lucky that swimming is so good for my fitness, health and well-being – things I truly value – but this is not the reason I do it. I swim because I can, because of how I feel in the water and because of how it leaves me feeling after I've swum.

I swim for different reasons at different times. In pools, I swim for fitness and to relax and unwind. Outdoors, I swim to connect with nature and the environment, for adventure, for the challenge of getting into cold water or covering a long distance. Sometimes I race. I almost always swim with friends, and frequently share coffee and cake with them afterwards.

Some of my earliest memories involve swimming. I remember the first time I swam without armbands, at about four years old, from the handrail on the steps to the wall in our local pool, a distance of 2 or 3 metres (2.2–3.3 yards). I swam with Cheltenham Swimming and Water Polo Club and then for my university team. I remember family holidays to Wales and Cornwall and playing in the sea, and day trips to old gravel pit lakes that had been made safe for swimming. In my 20s, I spent three years living and working in West Africa, where I frequently swam in the Gambia River and bodysurfed in the Atlantic.

Returning to London, I joined a masters swimming club and dabbled in triathlon, which gave me my first experiences of open water racing. Now, I'm lucky enough to live close to a safe spot on the Thames, which is ideal for both short winter dips and longer swims in summer.

In 2011, noticing the growth in popularity of open water events following the addition of marathon swimming to the Olympic programme in 2008, I saw a gap in the market for a dedicated magazine about outdoor swimming and launched *H2Open*, which we later rebranded to *Outdoor Swimmer*.

Swimming is a big part of my life. I think and write about swimming every day. It has helped keep me fit and healthy for more than 50 years, and it has allowed me to connect and make friends both locally and around the world. It has also helped me through bereavement and grief, and has taken me to places I would have never otherwise visited, and facilitated amazing adventures. It has given me confidence to try other activities, such as windsurfing, kayaking and stand up paddleboarding (SUP). It is an important part of who I am.

I love encouraging other people to swim outdoors and seeing the delight on their faces when they have an experience that exceeds their expectations, which it often does. I hope this book inspires you to try swimming in nature if you haven't done so already. And if you already swim outdoors, I hope it reveals new ideas and opportunities for you to explore as you continue your swimming journey.

As we say at *Outdoor Swimmer* magazine: swim wild and free.

SIMON GRIFFITHS

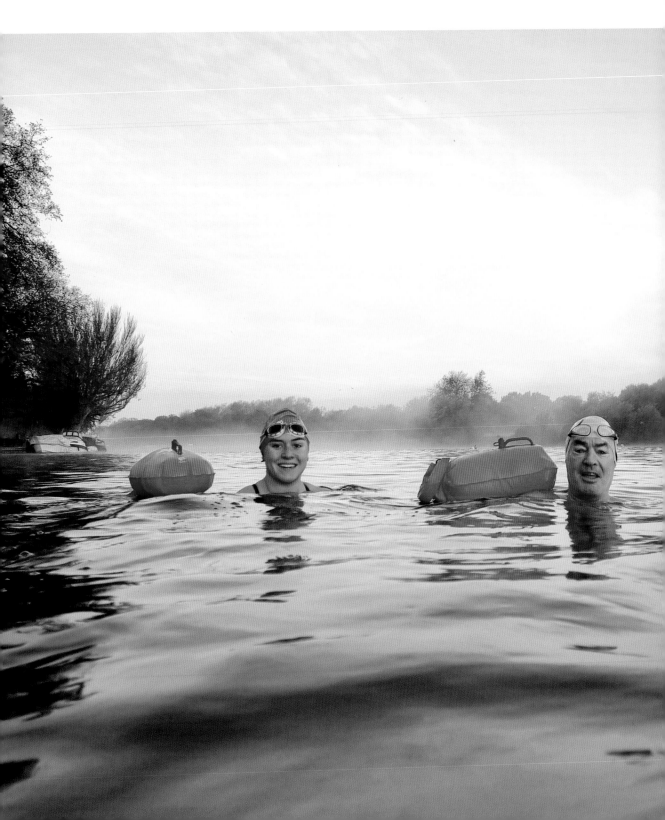

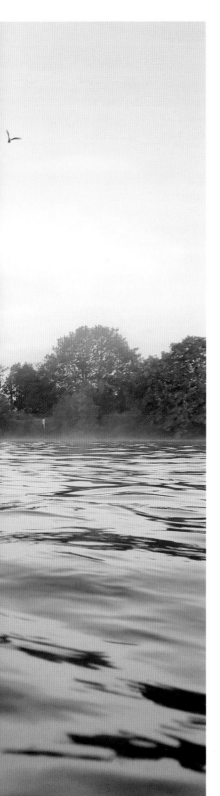

CHAPTER I

GETTING STARTED

What is outdoor swimming, why should you do it, how good a swimmer do you need to be and how do you get started? Also, find out why cold water isn't as big a barrier as you might think and how you can start swimming outdoors even in the middle of winter.

WHAT DO WE MEAN BY OUTDOOR SWIMMING?

Outdoor swimming offers something for everyone, from swimming in remote and untamed bodies of water to triathlon-style racing, long-distance challenges such as English Channel crossings and cold water dipping. I also include lidos, because they are special places. Other terms you may hear used are as follows.

Open water swimming
Usually in connection to events and racing, often in wetsuits, and training for these events.

Wild swimming
Meaning swimming in unsupervised locations in seas, estuaries, rivers, ponds, lochs and lakes.

Marathon swimming
This can refer either to the 10km (6.2-mile) marathon swim distance and Olympic distance open water event, or longer (typically solo) swims across large bodies of water, such as the English Channel or Catalina Channel.

Winter swimming and cold water swimming
This is swimming outside, in natural water temperatures in winter, either for recreation or in competition. This includes swimming in unheated outdoor pools.

Adventure swimming
This combines elements of wild and marathon swimming, often with a theme of exploration or a journey, and may take place over several days or longer.

> The broad definition of outdoor swimming is any swimming that takes place in water that isn't covered by a roof.

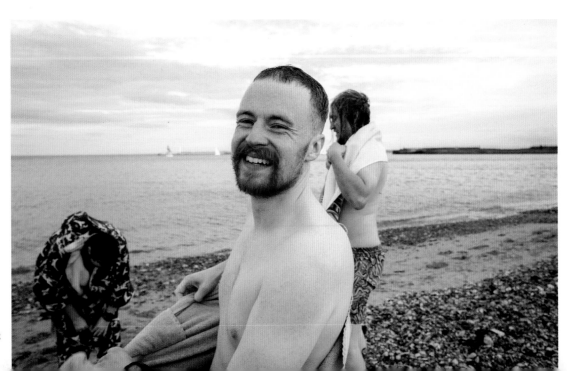

WHY SWIM OUTDOORS?

Walking across frosted grass in flip-flops, my toes go numb before I reach the water. In the early morning sun, mist rises from the Thames, giving an illusion of warmth. The water is, in fact, warmer than the air, but not by much, and it won't feel like it. Water sucks heat out of your body much quicker than air. I strip to my swimming costume, clip a bright orange float around my waist (so that the rowers will see me) and slide into the river. My breathing and heart rates immediately jump as the cold grips me. I try not to squeal and push aside the desire to jump straight back out. I swim slowly, with my head out of the water.

After around 90 seconds, something strange happens. I begin to feel comfortable, despite the temperature. I start to enjoy the sensation of cold water against my skin. This gives me chance to appreciate the beauty of the moment. The water is mirror-flat and still. A pair of swans glide by, close, but not threatening. A handful of tufted ducks circle, warily. Three Canada geese swoop in, honking, waterskiing briefly on their feet before settling on to the water. I look out for the kingfisher I spotted twice last summer, always hopeful of another glimpse of dazzling turquoise swooping across the water. I wonder if the local grey seal will make an appearance, half wanting it, and half fearing it. He's twice my size and I've seen what he can do to the fish he catches here. I swim over to the sunny side of the river. It always feels warmer there though it isn't really.

I don't stay in long. In early spring temperatures 10 minutes is plenty to get the benefits of a dip and I don't want to risk hypothermia.

Researchers say cold water immersion results in a surge in hormones that give you a natural mood boost. A refreshing early morning dip helps me tackle the day's work, including writing this book. Longer term, scientists at the University of Cambridge have proposed that regular swimming in cold water may reduce your risk of Alzheimer's. They discovered elevated levels of the protein RBM3 in regular cold water swimmers. In mice, this protein helps regenerate synapses in the brain.

In addition, there is a growing body of evidence showing that connecting with nature, and blue and green spaces, boosts your immediate health and well-being.

In a survey of swimmers carried out by *Outdoor Swimmer* magazine, 75 per cent of women and 68 per cent of men said that swimming outdoors was 'very important or essential' to their general sense of well-being. In addition, 73 per cent of women and 64 per cent of men said the same thing about their mental health, while the numbers for physical fitness were 62 per cent for women and 66 per cent for men.

Other highly rated benefits of outdoor swimming included a boost to confidence in other areas of life and an improved social life. When asked about the main reason they swim outside, around one-third said it was for their health and well-being, and around a fifth stated it was to connect with nature.

I am sure that as you explore outdoor swimming, you will experience these benefits for yourself and, in addition, find your own reasons to swim. (For links and further information on what the science says, please *see* Further reading and references on pp. 102–103.)

SWIMMING FOR ALL

People sometimes tell me they are not a good enough swimmer to swim outdoors. In most cases, this is nonsense. Swimming in natural waters does not require any special skills or abilities. If you can swim in a pool, or if you can float and propel yourself gently forwards or backwards, you can swim outdoors. In a way, the idea of being a 'good' outdoor swimmer doesn't make sense. Like walking, it's something you just do. It's more important to know how to stay safe and where to swim than to become a faster swimmer.

Of course, if you want to race, swim in difficult conditions or tackle a long-distance challenge, then you may want to improve your swimming skills, strength and fitness (and all of this is covered later). And many people starting out also benefit from refreshing their swimming abilities and testing their water confidence in the safe environment of a pool before venturing outside. But don't let 'I'm not a good enough swimmer' be the excuse that stops you exploring outdoor swimming.

The great thing about swimming outside is that all the health and well-being benefits just happen, whoever you are. All you need to do is get in the water and enjoy it. You don't need a training programme or goals or a target weight or a special diet. You just need to turn up. I've swum with people of all ages, shapes and sizes, from a wide range of ethnic groups, and with long-term physical and mental health conditions. The water doesn't discriminate.

Swimming outdoors in natural environments does, however, present practical difficulties for some swimmers with disabilities, primarily around access, but many still swim and enjoy all the benefits the activity provides. As part of my research, I spoke to several outdoor swimmers with disabilities and you will read about their experiences and passion for swimming in Chapter 5.

Finally, outdoor swimming can be a low-cost activity. There are no entry fees to swim in the sea or rivers, nor for many lakes or lochs. Kit is minimal. A wetsuit could cost you several hundred pounds if you choose to use one, but you don't have to (except at some commercial venues and events). Apart from that, unless you are skinny dipping, any old costume will do and everything else is optional.

With so much in its favour, you might be wondering what the downsides are. Luckily, unlike medication, there are no known side-effects to outdoor swimming. However, there are risks and hazards you need to be aware of and manage. These are covered in detail in Chapter 2.

In a survey, 50 per cent of swimmers with long-term conditions or disabilities say outdoor swimming brings them a lot of benefits, while a further 26 per cent say it's a complete game changer.

COME IN! THE WATER IS LOVELY

Perhaps the biggest barrier to people trying outdoor swimming for the first time is a fear of getting cold. I will let you into an outdoor swimmers' secret: there is no water that is too cold to swim in. None. Anywhere on this planet. You will, initially, find that hard to believe. But for now, trust me on this.

This doesn't mean you can blithely plunge into any body of water. You need to understand cold water shock and how to deal with the impact of immersion in cold water, which we cover in detail in Chapter 6. Most of us have been pampered by centrally heated homes and offices, and warm indoor pools. You need to re-wild yourself and accept that sometimes you may get cold. But not miserable.

I've met swimmers who prefer swimming outside in the winter to the summer and like getting cold. One-third of male swimmers and 45 per cent of female swimmers say that cold water never stops them swimming outside as much as they would like to, and fewer than 8 per cent of both men and women say the cold is a big worry.

You will, I assure you, adapt to swimming in cooler water and enjoy it.

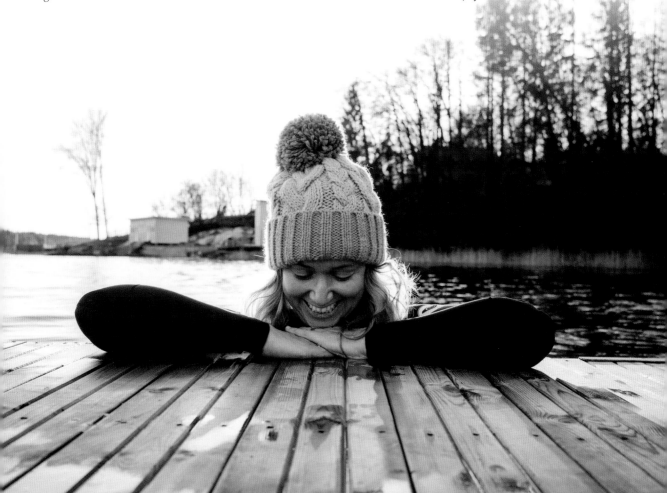

WHERE DO YOU START?

Getting started is often the hardest part and it's normal to be nervous. But I promise, it's worth facing your fears. You'll hear from many people through this book who will tell you that outdoor swimming has been life-changing for them, in a good way.

Health and Safety Check

1. Outdoor swimming is a very safe activity. But like any outdoor activity, it carries some risks. While it's unlikely something will go wrong, a mishap or miscalculation in open water could be fatal. It's therefore essential to familiarise yourself with the risks and how to manage them before you swim. The last thing I want is for readers of this book to end up being fearful of open water, but I can't overstress the importance of respecting it.

Before you embark on your outdoor swimmer journey, read through Chapter 2 and think about your safety, and that of anyone swimming with you, every time you swim.

2. For the unwary and inexperienced, cold water is the biggest threat. Immersion in cold water results in cold water shock, which provokes (among other things) an involuntary gasp response. If this happens when your face is underwater, you could inhale water, and one or two gasps can lead to drowning. The easy way to avoid this is to not put your face in the water until your breathing is under control, and never jump or dive in.

3. In addition, cold water immersion causes vasoconstriction, which means the heart needs to work harder. It also causes your heart rate to spike. When I first started swimming in cold water, I noticed that my heart rate would jump to between 150 and 160 beats per minute. This is a level I'd associate with hard exercise yet I was only stepping into cold water. People with underlying heart conditions should therefore check with a medical expert before attempting cold water swimming.

4. Finally, natural water can never be guaranteed free of pathogens and therefore may not be appropriate if you have a compromised immune system. If you have a health condition or any doubts, please take advice from your doctor before swimming outdoors, especially in water of less than 15ºC (59ºF).

For most people, though, the benefits far outweigh the risks, provided you swim sensibly and take appropriate precautions. Remember, respect the water, but don't fear it.

Swimmers with disabilities, chronic health conditions or mobility restrictions

Because of the support from the water, people with disabilities, chronic health conditions or mobility restrictions often find swimming more achievable than other outdoor activities. People suffering from chronic illness or recovering from serious health issues also often report pain relief and symptom alleviation as a result of swimming outdoors. However, access to the water can be difficult. My advice to all swimmers is to always plan your entry and exit in advance and make sure you will be able to leave the water when and where you want to. This is even more important if you have mobility restrictions. *See* pp. 86–88 for more on this.

Swim with Other People

There are people who love the peace and solitude of a lone swim, which I understand but do not recommend. Please try to find a group or someone else to swim with. Alternatively, ask a friend to paddle next to you in a kayak or on a SUP, or watch you from the bank.

Try searching Facebook for local outdoor swimming groups. There are hundreds around the world. Most will welcome new swimmers, show you places to swim and help you learn the basics. Alternatively, visit the Mental Health Swims (MHS) website and see if there is a Swim Host near you. MHS is a fantastic organisation offering a welcoming swim experience to anyone.

The only exceptions to the rule of never swimming alone are if you swim in lidos, at lifeguarded beaches or at supervised venues, where someone can assist you if you get into difficulties. These are all also great places to start your outdoor swimming journey, so let's take a brief look at each of those.

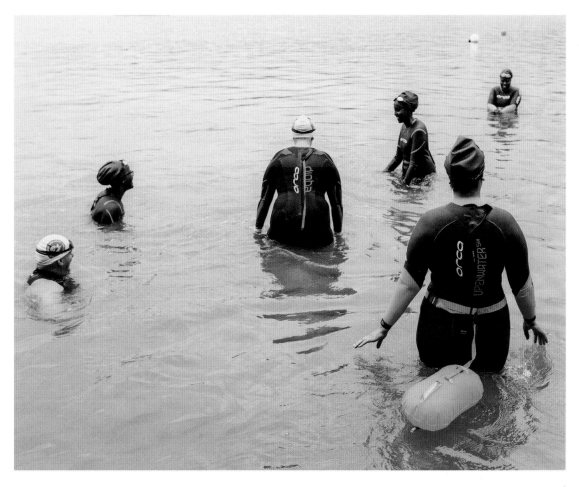

Lidos

I'm a massive fan of lidos and they are a fantastic stepping stone between indoor pools and the great outdoors. Growing up, I spent much of my summer holidays at my local lido. Back then, like many other outdoor pools, it was continually threatened with closure and it's wonderful to see lidos thriving today as part of a growing revival. I now frequently swim at a pool that was closed down in the 1980s and then rescued through community action.

Warm lidos combine the joys of swimming outside with the luxury of heated water. However, to prepare yourself for a true natural temperature experience, you may want to visit an unheated lido. Here, you can find out what it feels like to swim in cool water without the other factors that make rivers, lakes and oceans somewhat intimidating. The water is clean and clear, you can see and touch the bottom, and there are lifeguards if you need assistance. Lidos are brilliant places to build your swimming confidence. It's not essential you swim in one before venturing into open water, but I recommend it if you can.

If you swim in an unheated lido, especially in the cooler months of the year, remember to familiarise yourself with the risks of swimming in cold water (for more about this, *see* Chapter 6).

Lifeguarded Beaches

Every time I swim in the sea, it feels special. Living in London, I don't swim in the sea as often as I would like, but writing this inspired me to press gang my family into an impromptu day trip to a beach. The sea, however, presents several challenges for swimmers, which we'll cover in more detail later, in Chapter 3.

When you're starting out, head for a lifeguarded beach, swim in the area marked for swimming and only swim when the lifeguards put the safe swimming flags out.

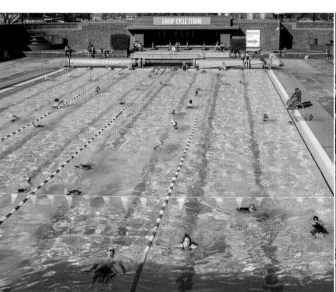

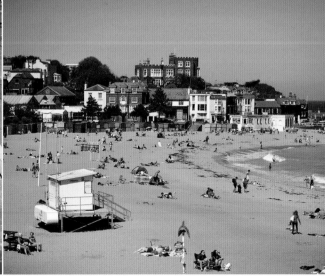

Swim parallel to the shore and consider staying within your depth if you are new to sea swimming. In general, it is easier to swim beyond the breakers, but playing in the surf is lots of fun, too.

The only exceptions to swimming in the sea at a lifeguarded beach for beginners might be if you're swimming with an experienced coach or guide or are joining an organised and responsible group.

> **Safety tip**
> Beaches are rarely lifeguarded throughout the year. The exact dates of lifeguard coverage vary by beach, so check before you go.

Supervised Venues

Supervised venues originally came about to serve the needs of triathletes, since an open water swim is a key feature in triathlon.

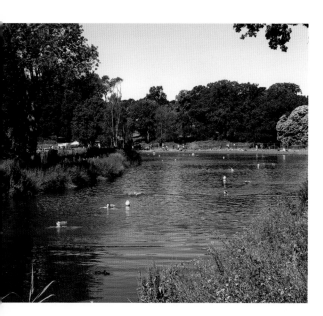

Their set-up and operation often reflects this. The majority of supervised venues are in private lakes. Typically, a swim route is marked out with brightly coloured buoys, which swimmers are expected to follow as they would in the race portion of a triathlon, in the direction specified. A circuit or loop often reflects standard triathlon distances of 400m (440 yards), 750m (820 yards) and sometimes 1500m (1640 yards).

As outdoor swimming has become more popular, the proportion of swimmers, rather than triathletes, using supervised venues has increased. In many places, swimmers now outnumber triathletes. Venues are making changes to reflect this, such as extending the swimming season into autumn and winter, and introducing shorter loops for beginners.

Good things about swimming at supervised venues include regular water quality checks and the presence of lifeguards, both on the water and watching from the side. Some venues offer introductory sessions and coaching, which makes them great places to start your outdoor swimming journey. I like that you can put your head down and swim at a supervised venue without the risk of being struck by another water user, which worries me when I swim in a busy river or the sea.

The main downsides are the requirement to follow a set course and the cost, typically £6 to £10 per swim in the UK. However, remember that you are paying for your safety and reassurance. Sometimes, opening hours are restricted and unsociable. Also, before you visit a venue, check their wetsuit policy. These may be compulsory or prescribed if the water temperature is below a certain level. Some venues now require swimmers to use a tow float.

YOUR FIRST SWIM: EASE YOURSELF IN GENTLY

Don't rush your first outdoor swimming experiences. You'll enjoy them more, and stay safer, if you start slowly.

Take your time to familiarise yourself with outdoor swimming. If you've only ever swum in pools, you will almost certainly find the water cold to start with, even with a wetsuit. There is no wall to hang on to and rest at. There are no black lines or tiles to follow to help you swim straight. You might not be able to see the bottom or have any idea how deep the water is. The unfathomable depth may unnerve you. That's OK. But from a swimming perspective, deep is better – there is less chance of swimming into anything, such as underwater plants or rocks. There might also be waves and currents.

All of these factors can be challenging to start with, but fun when you make use of them. You may need to swim outside several times before you start adapting to these differences and then a few more times to feel comfortable with them. Eventually, you will embrace and celebrate them, and you'll miss them the next time you swim in a pool.

1. Make your first swim short. A few minutes is plenty. Paddle or wade if you like, maybe dip your shoulders under the water. Swim a few strokes if you want to. There is no success or failure here.

2. Do what feels right, make it a positive experience, leave smiling and come back wanting more.

3. One thing that was drilled into me as a teenager doing lifesaving qualifications is to never dive into murky water, even in an emergency. You may end up as a casualty yourself if you hit a hidden object. Plus you may experience cold water shock.

4. Try to give yourself at least two minutes in the water on your first swim. That is enough time to get through the main impact of cold water shock and to start feeling more comfortable with the temperature. But don't be concerned if this feels unachievable. Try again another day.

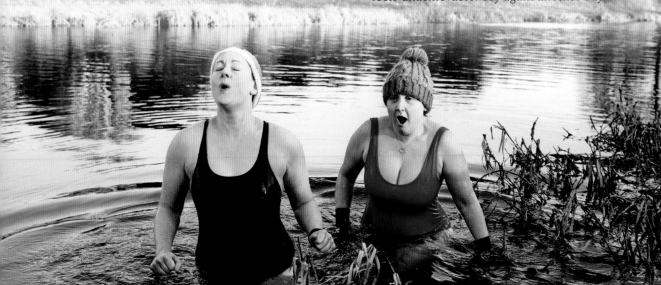

Can I start swimming outdoors in winter?

One of the biggest trends over the past few years in outdoor swimming is the growth in winter swimming. Swimming outdoors in winter isn't new. London's Serpentine Swimming Club has held a Christmas Day race since at least 1864. However, until relatively recently, winter swimming was a minority activity. No longer. According to a survey in 2020, 75 per cent of people who had recently taken up outdoor swimming planned to continue through the winter.

Outdoor waters in the northern hemisphere typically reach their peak in late summer. In Brighton, for example, the average sea temperatures in August and September range between around 16 and 19ºC (60.8–66.2ºF). Shallow lakes and ponds in Britain and northern Europe may reach 25ºC (77ºF), but more typically hover around 16–22ºC (60.8–71.6ºF). Going into autumn, inland lakes and rivers cool faster than the sea. Parts of the Thames can drop below 2ºC (35.6ºF) in January, while lakes and ponds sometimes freeze. In Brighton, the sea is coldest in February and March, bottoming out at around 6ºC (42.8ºF).

It's always worth checking your local temperatures and understanding how they vary. Some places have a much greater range than others. For example, the average sea temperature in Coney Island, New York, ranges from 4.4–23.4ºC (39.9–74.1ºF) while at La Jolla, California, the range is only 14.9–19.8ºC (58.8–67.6ºF).

In comparison, indoor pools generally keep the water at around 28–31ºC (82.4–87.8F). Even on a hot summer day, outdoor water will most likely be colder than what you're used to in a pool. Despite that, most people find summer water temperatures comfortable enough after a few swims. The usual advice, therefore, is to start your outdoor swimming journey in the summer. You can then keep swimming through the autumn and gradually acclimatise as the water cools.

But what if you're reading this in the winter? Can you start now? Yes, you can, but it will be more challenging than starting in the summer and there are additional safety considerations.

Tips for starting outdoor swimming in winter

- Read Chapter 6, on winter and cold water swimming (see pp. 90–105.)
- Familiarise yourself with the risks of cold water shock, swim failure and hypothermia.
- Swim with experienced winter swimmers who will support you.
- Swim at a supervised venue, such as an unheated lido or a commercial venue, while you learn the ropes.
- Don't be peer-pressured into staying in the water too long. Limit yourself to 10 minutes maximum for your first winter.
- If you feel like you have to get out immediately, that's OK. Come back another day and try again.
- Feel free to use neoprene accessories such as gloves, booties or a full wetsuit.

In other words, do everything you can to have a positive and safe experience. Remember, it's supposed to be fun, despite the cold, although it may take you a few swims to appreciate it. It's also fine if you find outdoor swimming in winter is not for you. There is no rule that says you have to swim in icy water to be a genuine outdoor swimmer. Come back in spring or summer when it's warmer.

What Stroke Should I Swim?

You can swim any officially recognised stroke you like or you can make up your own. When starting out, swim the stroke you are most comfortable with. I often hear people say: 'I need to learn front crawl.' If you want to, great. But you don't need to. The table below sets out some advantages and disadvantages to each stroke, in traditional individual medley order.

The pros and cons of different strokes

Stroke	Advantages	Disadvantages
Butterfly	Fun to swim Feels great if you can do it Looks impressive You can see where you're going	Exhausting* Can be splashy and disturbing Hard to learn
Backstroke	Relaxing Good for looking at the clouds or stars Keeps your face out of the water Best for floating and conserving energy	Hardest stroke to see where you're going Not allowed in some events or at some venues**
Breaststroke	Most people find it easy Best for taking in the scenery and observing nature Best for swimming and chatting You can keep your face out of the water	Difficult to swim in a wetsuit Can strain your neck Slowest stroke
Front crawl	Fastest stroke Most efficient stroke for long distances Relaxing when you get the timing right Most popular stroke at events and races	Need to look up frequently to see where you're going Your face is always in the water You can't chat while swimming

* Some people swim long-distance butterfly. In 2002, Julie Bradshaw set a new record of 14 hours 18 minutes for swimming across the English Channel using butterfly.

**At events and venues, swimmers needing assistance are advised to roll on to their backs and wave for help. People swimming backstroke might be confused with people needing help.

If you're confident in the water and can propel yourself through it, then that is good enough to get started. Speed isn't an issue in still water. At the Great North Swim one year, I watched two women completing the mile in just under two hours. They'd spent the whole time swimming head-up breaststroke, chatting and enjoying the view. The fastest swimmers put their heads down and powered around the course in about 20 minutes. They didn't stop to talk and barely had time to admire the mountains surrounding the lake. Tell me who got the best value for money?

MY STORY

Swimming clears my mind

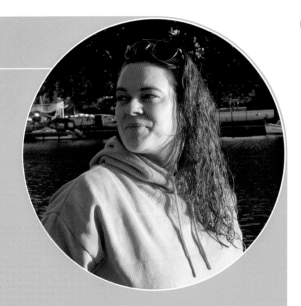

I could swim, but only in the sense that if you chucked me in a pool, I would be able to get back to the side. When my friend Gina took me to Chertsey Meads for my first outdoor swim, I freaked out so much I was barely able to get to the other side of the river. Six training swims later I found myself climbing into the Thames for the Henley Swim Pub to Club mile.

The prospect of swimming so far was too enormous and as I watched the others swim off, I panicked. I was immobilised and wanted to get out. I wanted to cry. But somehow I managed to force my face into the murky water and start swimming. Forty minutes later, I had completed the mile and I was officially hooked. I now swim as often as I can in the river, even in the winter, when the temperature is less than 5ºC (41ºF) and the current is fierce.

I find that when I swim, my awareness will shift from whatever is going on in my head to what my body is sensing. As I swim towards the horizon, I become aware of the sounds of the river and the way the water feels as I move through it. Minute changes in my surroundings are observed. Even in winter, when all you can do is swoosh, it is difficult to not appreciate the force of the flow of freezing water that burns your skin, carrying you along. In the water, my mind clears. Things that used to panic me now bring me peace.

Living and working in London, it is difficult to find the tranquillity outdoor swimming creates and, for me, time in the river has become vital.

VICKY MONTAG

This is just the beginning

This chapter has merely rippled the surface of what outdoor swimming can offer you. If you stick with it, you'll encounter adventures and experiences you never imagined. Swimming also gives you a means to exercise at almost any age, and a lifetime supply of self-administered health and well-being support. It may even help you find a job or new career. We will explore these topics in more detail through this book. Are you ready?

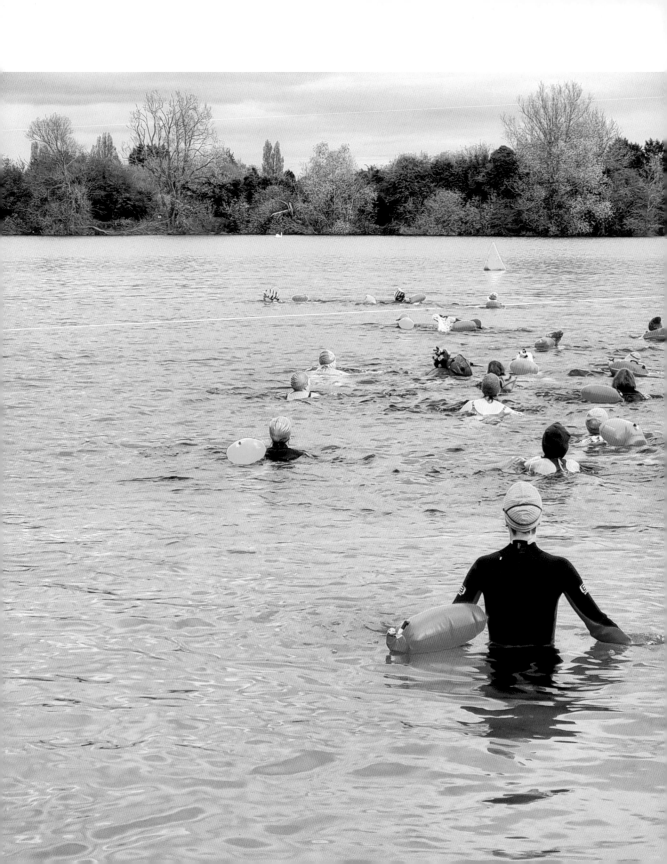

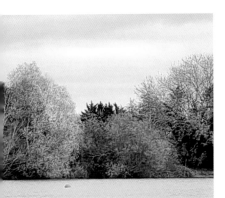

CHAPTER 2

STAYING SAFE

Outdoor swimming, and wild swimming in particular, takes you into the natural environment and exposes you to risks you might not encounter in daily life. Every pond, lake, beach or river is different, and the conditions change each time you swim. The key to staying safe is planning and judgement. Each time you swim, ask yourself what are the hazards and how can you minimise the risks. This chapter shows you how to do this.

THINK BEFORE YOU SWIM

Water, while essential for life, and amazing for our health and well-being, can also kill us. Therefore, every time you swim, you must ensure you do it safely.

Data from the WAter Incident Database (WAID) shows that more than 300 people die each year in the UK from drowning. Globally, 372,000 people lose their lives to drowning each year. Despite this, with planning and experience, outdoor swimming is a safe activity, but you need to be aware of the risks and hazards, and prepare accordingly.

A closer look at the drowning statistics reveals that for nearly half of deaths, the person had no intention of being in the water. Walking and running account for nearly twice as many drowning deaths than swimming. The National Water Safety Forum (NWSF) put the risk of drowning while participating in watersports on a par with cycling or being a passenger in a car. In addition, they say: 'Fatal incidents at managed mass participation events and during supervised or coached scenarios are very rare.'

Top safety tips

- Respect the water.
- Never mix swimming and alcohol.
- Check your entry and exit points, taking into account currents and tides.
- Swim with other people. If you can, find experienced swimmers who are familiar with the swim spot.
- Don't jump or dive in. Enter the water slowly to prevent cold water shock or collision with hidden submerged objects.
- Let people know where you are, what you're doing and when you plan to return.
- Make sure you're visible in the water. Wear a brightly coloured cap and use a tow float.
- If someone gets in trouble, don't put yourself at risk. Call the emergency services for help.

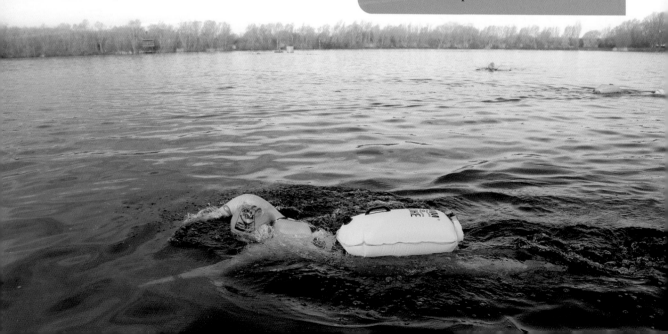

COPING WITH COLD

Natural water temperatures are almost always cooler than those of indoor heated swimming pools. Once you have adapted, the feeling of swimming in cool water is one of the many delights of outdoor swimming. But cold water can be dangerous because of cold water shock, autonomic conflict, swim failure and hypothermia. Researchers say cold water shock is responsible for a significant portion of drownings, so pay attention to this section.

Cold water shock

Cold water shock is your body's initial and automatic response to a rapid cooling in skin temperature resulting from immersion in water that's colder than you are accustomed to. Cold water is generally defined as water below 15ºC (59ºF), but some people may experience cold water shock at warmer temperatures than this. The response is immediate and involuntary, and causes a sharp intake of breath, an increase in breathing and heart rates, and an increase in blood pressure. It can also induce a feeling of panic. The cold water shock response only lasts a couple of minutes.

The good thing about the cold water shock response is that your body adapts to it quickly. About five or six immersions will significantly reduce the response. That's why you see experienced swimmers stepping into cold lakes as easily as they might slip into a hot tub. However, if you go into colder water than you've adapted to, you will again experience cold water shock.

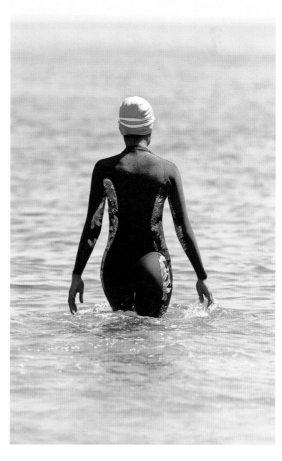

Minimise the risk
- Enter the water slowly but purposefully.
- Some people splash water on their face and neck as they find this reduces the impact.
- Keep your head above the water to ensure you don't inhale water.
- Wait until you can breathe calmly before moving out of your depth and attempting to swim.
- Understanding what is happening to your body will help you deal with it.

Autonomic Conflict

In a 2012 research paper in the *The Journal of Physiology* Michael Shattock and Michael Tipton proposed 'autonomic conflict' as a possible cause of death in swimmers. They noted that 67 per cent of drownings occur in strong swimmers and 55 per cent within 3m (3.3 yards) of a safe haven. As noted above, cold water shock causes an increase in heart rate. However, in mammals, including humans, a second phenomenon – the mammalian dive response – occurs. The diving response is triggered partly by breath holding and by the immersion of the face in cold water, and signals the heart to slow down to conserve oxygen, hence prolonging the dive time.

These two involuntary responses are in conflict (hence 'autonomic conflict') and the hypothesis is that this could trigger a potentially fatal arrhythmia. In a separate paper in the *British Journal of Sports Medicine* (2013), Professor Tipton suggested this may be the cause of some of the 30 deaths that occurred in the swim portion of triathlons in the USA between 2003 and 2011.

Minimise the risk
- While autonomic conflict deaths are rare, they emphasise the need to allow the cold water shock response to subside before immersing the face or holding your breath.
- This is especially important in events where the excitement of the race will also elevate your heart rate.

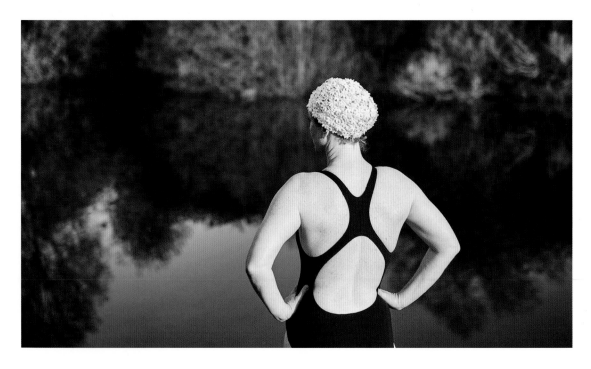

Swim Failure

When swimming, your body loses heat to the water. The colder the water, the faster the heat loss. The initial cooling affects the skin and results in cold water shock. The next stage in the cooling process affects superficial muscle and nerves, with the arms being particularly susceptible. This cooling weakens the muscle and may eventually lead to a point where you can no longer swim or use your arms to help you float, which results in swim failure.

How long this takes depends on multiple factors, including the water temperature and your body's size and shape. English Channel swimmers can swim for hours, without a wetsuit, in water temperatures between 14–18°C (57.2–64.4°F), without suffering swim failure. In icy water, swim failure may occur in less than 10 minutes.

Minimise the risk
- The key to avoiding swim failure is to be aware of the risk and the conditions, and to leave the water if you feel yourself slowing down or struggling to swim.
- If you notice that someone you're swimming with has suddenly lost speed or that their arms are moving slowly, they should get out and warm up.

Hypothermia

The longer you stay in cold water, the more heat your body loses. Your body attempts to minimise heat loss from the core by restricting blood flow to the extremities, which cool much faster. At some point – again determined by multiple factors including body morphology, fitness levels and water conditions – your core body temperature starts to drop. Studies show there is widespread variation between individuals, with some being able to stay in thermal equilibrium in cool water for several hours, because of the heat they are generating through exercising, and others becoming hypothermic within 30 minutes.

Typical normal body temperature is around 37°C (98.6°F). There isn't much margin as mild hypothermia starts at 35°C (95°F). Symptoms include shivering, apathy, fatigue and – importantly – impaired judgement. Someone with hypothermia might not realise it is happening.

Getting a little cold might be good for us. Getting very cold certainly isn't.

Minimise the risk
- Start with short swims to learn what your limits are.
- Always swim with other people.
- If your stroke rate slows down or you start to shiver, get out and warm up.
- You cannot use will power to prevent hypothermia nor can you simply ignore it and hope it passes.

My worst experience of hypothermia happened while swimming a length of Windermere. The water temperature was something like 13–15ºC (55.4–59ºF) and the swim took me nearly six hours. I don't have any memory of the final part of the swim. My last clear memory was stopping for a snack about four hours into the swim, shivering violently but determined to continue. The next thing I remember is lying in a tent, wrapped in multiple blankets and sleeping bags with someone trying to get me to drink warm, sweet, milky tea and telling me to stay awake. A short while later, an ambulance arrived and took me to hospital where they stuck me under an infrared lamp for several hours. I was lucky to make a complete and rapid recovery; severe hypothermia can lead to cardiac arrest.

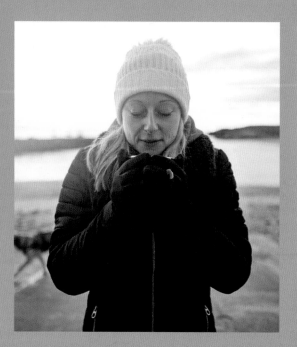

Continued Cooling or 'Afterdrop'

Cooling of the body is primarily a conduction phenomenon, with the extremities and surfaces of the body affected first. The cold steadily spreads to your core. Once you leave the water, the cold continues to spread from the cooler parts of your body to the core. Measurements of core body temperature using a rectal thermometer show it can continue to drop for 20–30 minutes after swimming. Swimmers refer to this phenomenon as 'afterdrop', while scientists prefer the term 'continued cooling'.

In practice, this means that you could be fine when leaving the water, but hypothermic 20 minutes later. It is why winter swimmers often start to shiver 10–20 minutes after they have finished swimming, despite dressing quickly in multiple layers of warm clothes.

Minimise the risk
- Leave the water before you get too cold.
- Dress quickly, starting with the top half of your body.
- Keep out of the wind.
- Sipping a warm drink helps psychologically more than physiologically, but it's worth doing for comfort.
- Intense exercise is best avoided, but brisk walking can help.
- You shouldn't attempt to drive, ride a bike or operate machinery until you have properly rewarmed.

Raynaud's phenomenon

According to Scleroderma & Raynaud's UK (SRUK), a charity dedicated to improving the lives of people affected by these conditions, for people with Raynaud's: 'Hands, feet, fingers or toes are over-sensitive to even the slightest changes in temperature, cold conditions and sometimes emotional stress.'

When Raynaud's is triggered, the fingers typically turn white (or paler, for people with dark skin) and numb. Later, during recovery, they can turn reddish or purple and can become painful.

Swimming outdoors sometimes involves exposure to cold. We know, through swimmer surveys, that people who are affected by Raynaud's in daily life tend to be affected when they swim. We also know that outdoor swimming triggers similar symptoms in some people who are not normally affected by Raynaud's.

In most cases, symptoms are nothing more than temporary numbness, a little bit of discomfort and awkwardness, and some entertainment as the fingers change colour. Recovery is normally swift and blood flow to the extremities resumes once your core has rewarmed. Unfortunately, for some people, the condition causes considerable pain. If this happens to you, seek medical advice. Luckily, the condition rarely prevents people from swimming.

It's possible, but not known, that suffering from Raynaud's could make you more susceptible to non-freezing cold injury, which is more serious and could result in permanent damage. For most swimmers, repeated triggering of symptoms should not cause any worsening of the condition or any long-term damage.

> **Minimise the risk**
> - You may be able to reduce or prevent symptoms by wearing neoprene socks and gloves, and limiting the time you spend in cold water.
> - Ensure you dress and warm up quickly after swimming.
> - Put on gloves after swimming.

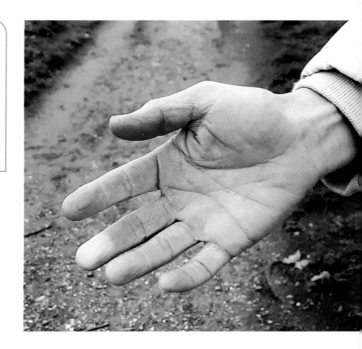

Non-Freezing Cold Injury

Non-freezing cold injury is a poorly understood condition that can affect extremities – usually fingers or toes – that have been exposed to the cold. What we do know has mostly been learned through observations of military personnel, although it has also been reported in outdoor swimmers. It is usually associated with extreme-cold swimming (below 5ºC/41ºF), but may affect some people after prolonged exposure at warmer temperatures. Studies in the military suggest it may affect people of African descent more than white people.

In the initial stages, the extremities lose feeling and turn pale. On rewarming, the skin can turn mottled blue (which may be difficult to see on darker skin) while the numbness persists. This stage can last from a few hours to several days until it is replaced by swelling, redness and pain accompanied by fingertip numbness. Blistering and permanent tissue damage can occur. The swelling can last for several weeks or even years.

Some restriction of blood flow to the extremities is normal when swimming in cold water and is not a cause for panic or concern. The initial symptoms of non-freezing cold injury look similar to those of Raynaud's, which is widespread but does not cause any permanent harm.

Minimise the risk
- Always rewarm the hands and feet slowly to prevent chilblains.
- If you find your extremities react more to the cold than those of the people you swim with or the numbness persists for a prolonged period after swimming, consider taking precautions such as wearing neoprene gloves (*see* Chapter 7) in cooler conditions.
- Avoid extended exposure to extreme cold.

Won't a wetsuit protect me from the cold?

A wetsuit adds a layer of thermal protection and enables you to stay in the water longer and be comfortable at cooler temperatures. However, a wetsuit does not protect you from cold water shock as water has to come into your wetsuit for it to work properly. For the inexperienced, a wetsuit can magnify the sense of panic induced by cold water shock due to its tightness around the chest and neck. Autonomic conflict is also still a risk. Therefore, follow the same precautions for entering the water whether you are wearing a wetsuit or not. Because it slows the rate of cooling, a wetsuit reduces the extent of afterdrop.

For more on wetsuits, their benefits and how to choose the right one for swimming, *see* Chapter 7.

NB: You can still get cold and become hypothermic in a wetsuit.

Hyperthermia

While rare in open water swimming, it is possible to overheat in certain conditions. Hyperthermia and heatstroke are believed to be the cause of, or a contributing factor in, the death of elite marathon swimmer Fran Crippen, who disappeared in 2010 during a 10km (6.2-mile) swimming race in Abu Dhabi. His body was found two hours later. He was 26 years old. The water temperature at the time was more than 30ºC (86ºF).

In recreational swimmers, overheating is more likely in cooler but still warm conditions and when wearing a wetsuit. Consider swimming without a wetsuit on those rare occasions when the water temperature exceeds 24ºC (75.2ºF). If you must wear the wetsuit, keep your swim short and flush water through the wetsuit frequently by tugging gently at the neck to let water in.

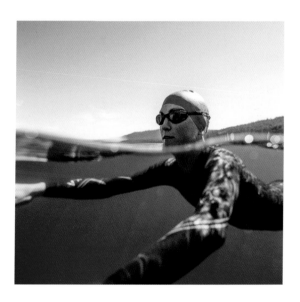

Swimming-Induced Pulmonary Oedema

Swimming-induced pulmonary oedema (SIPE) is a rare condition you should be aware of as a swimmer, especially if you do long-distance swims. SIPE occurs when fluid from the pulmonary capillaries leaks into the air sacs and results in a shortness of breath that is disproportionate to the effort you put in, during or immediately after swimming. Other symptoms may include coughing and coughing up phlegm or bloody fluid, whistling or crackling noises from the chest and a feeling of tightness around the chest. Symptoms usually reduce when the swimmer is back on land.

If you suspect you or someone you are with is suffering from SIPE then get out of the water immediately and call for medical assistance. It could be life-threatening if you continue swimming.

We do not know what causes SIPE, but risk factors may include high blood pressure, being female, being aged over 40, a tight-fitting wetsuit, over-hydration, long-distance swims, lack of warm-up and a high level of exertion. Water inhalation is not believed to be a factor.

SIPE is rare. I only know of a handful of cases, but it's another good reason for never swimming alone. If you are unfortunate enough to need medical assistance with symptoms that may be SIPE, make sure that whoever is treating you knows you have been swimming in open water and considers SIPE as a diagnosis as the treatment is different than for water inhalation. If recognised and treated promptly, most cases resolve within 48 hours.

COPING WITH DIFFERENT WATER CONDITIONS

Part of the wonder and the challenge of swimming in the wild is experiencing and coping with the changing conditions. Whether it's the open sea, rivers or lakes, knowing how to cope will enhance your enjoyment.

Tides and Currents

Developing an appreciation of tides and their effects is an important skill for anyone contemplating swimming in the sea or tidal rivers. Tides can result in huge changes in water level and create strong currents.

The world's highest tides are found in Canada's Bay of Fundy, where the water level can change almost 16m (52.5ft). On the opposite side of the Atlantic, the UK also has some of the largest tidal ranges in the world. The water level in the Severn Estuary can change by as much as 15m (49.2ft) over the course of six hours – that's about three double decker buses stacked on top of each other. This change generates ferocious currents and rapidly submerges beaches. Your planned exit point could be deep underwater or high out of reach if you get your timing wrong. Always seek local knowledge before attempting to swim anywhere tidal.

In the English Channel, the tide causes currents to run roughly parallel to the shore. On an incoming tide, water moves up the Channel from the west. When the tide changes, the current reverses direction. If you look at the route a swimmer takes across the English Channel, you'll see that rather than swimming directly across, they follow a long, sweeping curve as they are first swept in one direction and then the other.

Different beaches have their own patterns and timings. If you plan to swim along a shoreline, make sure you know which way the current is flowing and when it will change.

It's easy to get caught out by tidal currents. Once, while swimming off a beach in West Africa, I stopped paying attention. When I looked up, I saw I had drifted 100m (110 yards) or so along the shore in just a couple of minutes. Not much, you might think. However, it would have been suicidal to attempt to swim directly back to shore as, at the point where I'd drifted to, the breakers were smashing over sharp rocks. I had to swim the 100m (110 yards) back again, against the current, to where I could safely get out of the sea on to the sandy beach. It was some of the hardest swimming I've ever done and I had to fight against a rising sense of panic. Obviously I made it, otherwise I wouldn't be here to write this, but as there were no lifeguards it could have had a much worse ending.

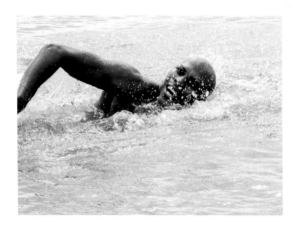

Rip Currents

Whereas tidal currents are reasonably predictable, rip currents are less so and therefore potentially more dangerous. Rip currents occur when the water from waves crashing on the beach sweeps back to sea through a narrow channel such as a break in a sandbar below the surface. The current stream may only be 10m (32.8ft) across, but it can quickly carry an unwary swimmer tens of metres/yards away from the shore in a short space of time. Avoid rip currents if you can.

At supervised beaches, lifeguards will be on the lookout for rips and will steer bathers away. However, if you do find yourself dragged away from the beach, stay calm. Instead of trying to swim against the current directly back to shore, take yourself out of it by swimming sideways first. Once you are out of the rip, you can swim back to the beach.

Undertow

Undertow is a different phenomenon to a rip current. Undertow happens continuously along the length of a beach where waves are crashing in. As the water slides back down the beach it slips under the next wave coming in, so the water underneath is moving in a different direction to that on top. This can unbalance you and knock you off your feet, but won't pull you out to sea like a rip current. If this happens, stay calm and wait for the next wave to carry you back up the beach.

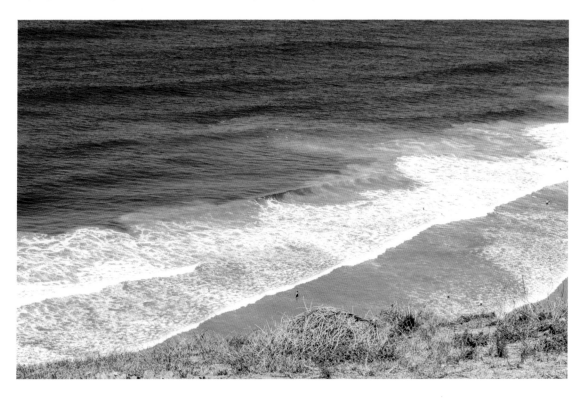

Rivers

Pay attention to currents in rivers. Generally and obviously, the current flows downstream. In straight sections, it tends to be faster in the middle and slower towards the edges. Where the river bends, the current sweeps around the outside and is slower on the inside. This often results in the river being deeper on the outside of the bend and shallower on the inside.

Obstacles in the water, such as boulders, fallen trees or bridge piers, can cause eddies or reversals in the current. It's worth spending time watching rivers and noticing these things. An awareness of how currents behave can help you to avoid dangers. You can also use your knowledge to your advantage.

Even a gentle current makes a big difference to how easily you can swim up or downstream. If you plan to use the same exit and entry points for a river swim, head upstream to start with so you can drift back with the flow when you want to finish. Keep clear of fallen branches and other obstacles in the water when river swimming as a fast current could pin you against them or even pull you under them.

In tidal rivers and estuaries, the direction of current reverses roughly every six hours and water flows upstream. Rivers can be tidal for a considerable distance inland. The Thames, for example, is tidal up to Teddington Lock, which is around 68 miles (110km) from where the river joins the sea. Always check the tide times to avoid being caught out by a change in current direction.

Some rivers have dams and reservoirs, and the flow downstream of these is controlled. Sometimes, additional water is released from the dam, which results in a rapid increase in the current.

Do your research before you swim, check the conditions when you arrive and take advice from local swimmers.

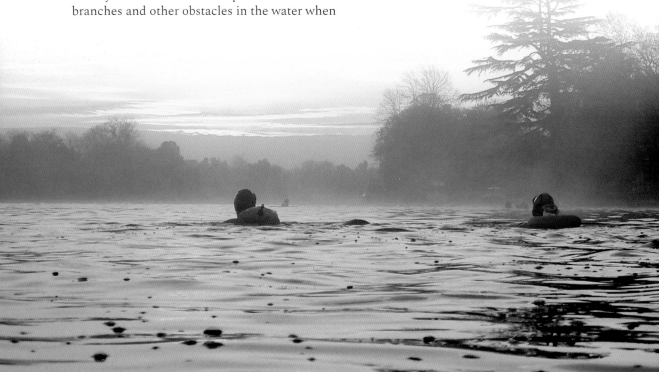

OTHER HAZARDS AND THINGS TO BE AWARE OF

As well as more obvious hazards, such as currents, like any activity in nature, wild swimming has its share of less visible risks that you should be aware of.

Cramp

Swimmers occasionally experience cramp, when certain muscles go into spasm. It most commonly affects the lower limbs and can be painful and disabling. If it happens while you're swimming in open water, it can be frightening and may cause you to panic. Some people are more prone to cramp than others. If you are such a person, you may have some experience of what triggers cramps and can try to avoid them. For example, if your legs are tired from running or cycling, they may be more likely to cramp up when swimming. One thing that causes my legs to cramp is if I try to sprint at the end of a long swim and kick too hard.

If you get cramp while swimming and it's preventing you from continuing, try rolling on to your back and floating. If you're wearing a wetsuit, you will float easily. If you can relax, it may ease off on its own. If not, wave one arm in the air with your fist clenched (so it's not mistaken for a friendly wave) and shout for assistance.

Cramp is another good reason to always swim with someone else. If you have a tow float (again, strongly recommended), you can rest on that temporarily. Some people also carry emergency floats that can be inflated from a CO_2 cartridge in seconds.

> You can't guarantee you will never get cramp while swimming, but you can ensure you're prepared to deal with it.

Stitch

You were probably told as a child not to swim within two hours of eating a big meal in case you got stitch. While the exact causes of stitch – or exercise-related transient abdominal pain in medical parlance – aren't fully understood, it does seem to be more prevalent after food, particularly if washed down with fizzy drinks. While it's unpleasant, and may cause you to slow down in a race or on a hard training session, it shouldn't disrupt a leisurely swim. Follow the same safety precautions as for cramp.

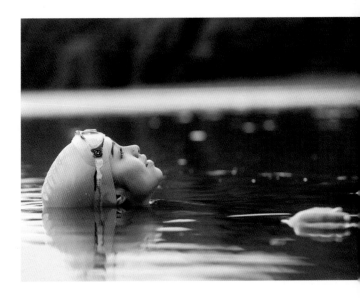

Cuts and Bruises

Acute physical injuries are rare in outdoor swimming, but do watch out for your feet when getting into and out of the water. A sharp stone can give you a nasty cut, and it's easy to stumble and hurt yourself on slippery or uneven rocks. I've also encountered broken glass and rusty bits of iron at swimming spots.

In the sea, be aware that waves can be powerful and could knock you off your feet, dump you on the beach or drag you into rocks. Coral reefs, while visually stunning, often have sharp edges. Coral cuts can leave traces of animal protein in the wound, which increases the chance of infection, so take care around them.

If you do cut yourself, it's best to get out of the water and clean the injury as soon as possible with drinking-quality running water to reduce the risk of infection. Minor cuts can usually be treated at home in the normal way but if you have any sign of infection, seek medical advice. For larger cuts, wounds with jagged edges or those that are contaminated with dirt, get immediate medical attention. You may need antibiotics or an injection to prevent tetanus.

The best way to avoid a mishap is to be choosy where you swim and pay attention to potential hazards. Wearing neoprene socks can help protect your feet and are a good option in some scenarios.

On holiday once, when I was young and reckless, I ran into the sea and threw myself into a dive once the water reached my thighs, and landed on a sharp rock a few centimetres below the surface. I was lucky it hit my stomach and not my face, and I got away with a minor gash and a faint scar. It was an important reminder of an essential safety precaution: never jump or dive into unknown water.

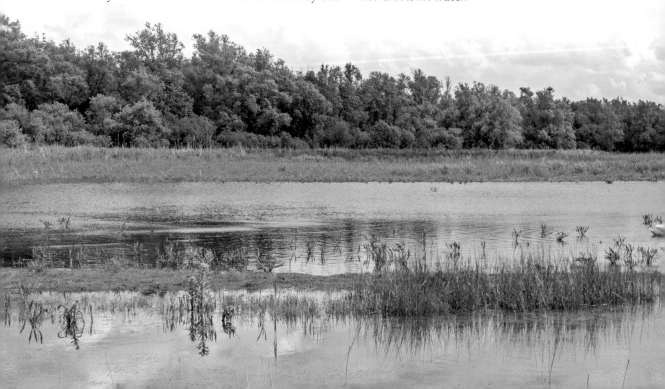

Weeds

Despite swimming outdoors for years, I still get moments of panic when I swim into aquatic plants, although it's irrational. I've heard many swimmers worrying about getting tangled in weeds and pulled down. Plants don't pull you down, but it sometimes feels as if the tendrils are looping around your ankles and tugging you under.

Shallow lakes are particularly prone to plant growth and can become choked with them in late summer. Some commercial venues actively clear the growth or put a special blue dye in the water that restricts their growth. Avoid swimming into weedy patches as it's unpleasant when they wrap around your arms and slow you down. If you do get tangled, calmly extract yourself, rather than flailing madly. Wearing a wetsuit or having a tow float to hold on to will help reduce panic or fears of being pulled down.

Once you get over any fear of aquatic plants, take some time to admire them.

Blue-Green Algae

Cyanobacteria (so named because of their blue colour) occur naturally in inland waters, estuaries and the sea. Normally, they are nothing to worry about and are an important part of aquatic ecosystems. However, under certain conditions they can reproduce rapidly, resulting in blue-green algae blooms. These blooms can quickly cover a large surface area and release toxins into the water. Not all blooms are toxic, but you can't tell by looking, so it's best to avoid swimming through them. Blooms affect the colour and clarity of the water, may look like paint on the surface and can produce scums. If in doubt, stay out. Also, algae bloom toxins can be fatal to dogs, so keep your pets out of the water too.

Blooms are a natural phenomenon but can be made worse by pollution, especially from fertilizers that can be washed off farmland by heavy rain.

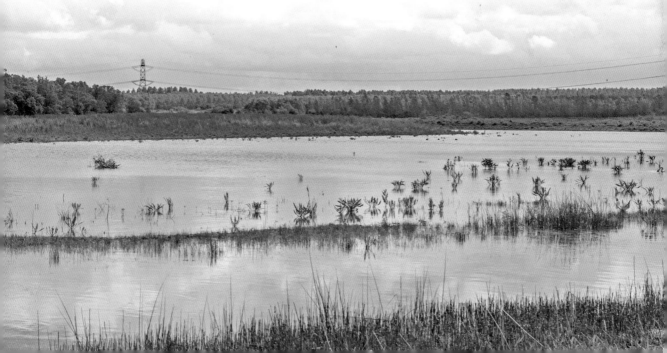

Weil's Disease

Weil's disease is the name given to a severe case of leptospirosis, a bacterial infection (caused by bacteria called leptospira) that is spread by animals and can affect people. You can catch it through contact with soil or water that's been contaminated by urine from affected animals. The majority of cases are related to agricultural work.

Public Health England says that cases of leptospirosis in the UK are rare and there is no reason why people shouldn't swim in open water because of it. However, it's worth being aware of it. If you experience flu-like symptoms after swimming, let your doctor know you have been exposed to open water and to consider Weil's disease as a possible diagnosis.

Other Waterborne Diseases

The sad reality is that sewage is routinely dumped in our rivers. Data from the Environment Agency shows sewage spilled into English waters from storm overflows 403,171 times in 2020. On top of that, our rivers, lakes and oceans are polluted by agricultural run-off. Luckily, the growth in outdoor swimming is increasing pressure on the government and water companies to reduce pollution, and I urge you to support any relevant campaigns to reduce this horror.

On a more positive note, I (along with many people I know) frequently swim in rivers, lakes and the sea, and rarely complain about any ill effects. Event organisers carry out independent tests of water quality in various bodies of water and would not be able to proceed if it didn't meet bathing water standards. Nevertheless, even without sewage and run-off, swimming in natural waters always carries some risk or waterborne diseases.

As a general precaution, avoid swallowing the water you're swimming in, don't swim if you have any open cuts, avoid swimming after heavy rain due to run-off and potential sewage spills, wash your hands as soon as you can after swimming and don't eat or drink anything until you have. Ask other swimmers about their preferred places to swim and if there are spots you should avoid. If you swim at supervised venues, they should be carrying out regular water quality tests. Designated bathing waters are monitored weekly through the summer.

In 2012, I took part in a river swimming race. Twenty-four hours later I had an unpleasant dose of diarrhoea and vomiting that lasted a couple of days. A subsequent investigation by Public Health England found that about one-third of the participants experienced similar symptoms, with four people admitted overnight to hospital. The event had taken place after heavy rain, which is believed to have washed sewage into the river, although the exact cause was never identified.

If you are unlucky enough to get ill because of swimming, most likely it will be mild and pass quickly, but obviously seek medical advice if you're worried.

Swimmer's Itch

There isn't a nice way to describe this. Swimmer's itch is caused by an allergic reaction to a tiny parasitic worm that burrows into your skin if you swim in infected water. It looks like an insect bite and can last (and itch) for several days. In severe cases, the itching causes significant discomfort and may prevent you from sleeping. On a more positive note, the parasite can't live in humans and can't enter your blood stream or deeper tissues. Its intended targets are waterfowl as part of a life cycle that also involves a stage in water snails. It is most prevalent in shallow, fresh water and tends to increase in warmer water.

Some swimmers are more affected than others. You can minimise the risk of infection by keeping to deeper water away from water plants that may harbour snails. A wetsuit will give you some protection, too.

If you do get infected, try not to scratch as this can cause infection. Instead, treat with anti-itch lotion. Over-the-counter antihistamines may help relieve symptoms if they are preventing you from sleeping. A cold compress may also give some relief, but a hot shower or bath may make it worse. While it sounds disgusting, there is no lasting harm.

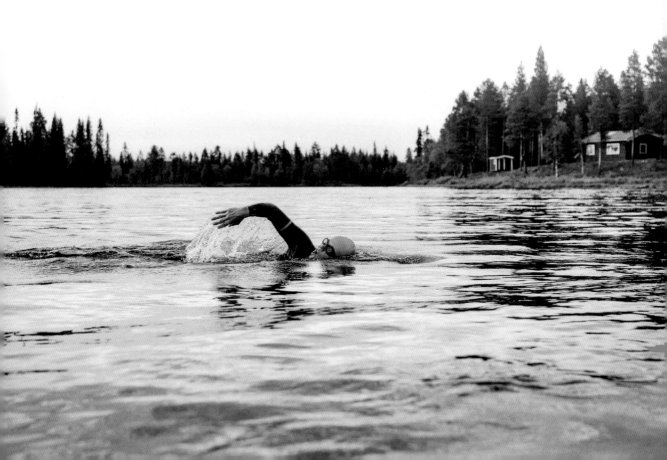

Boats and Other Water Users

Remember, swimmers aren't the only water users. Where I swim, I share the water with rowers, scullers, kayakers, dragon boaters, barges, party boats, day-hire boats, paddleboarders, sailors, punters and anglers. As a swimmer, you are the most vulnerable and least visible person on or in the water. Rowers and scullers both travel backwards. Larger boats, especially those steered from the rear, have a limited field of vision. Inexperienced (and occasionally inebriated) people in hire boats often don't look where they are going and pay little heed to navigational rules.

Despite these many hazards, I still see swimmers bobbing about, on their own, in the middle of the river or far from shore at sea, without any attempt to make themselves visible. Please don't do this.

If you can, swim in designated boat-free areas. When you share the water with other users, you must pay attention and choose the safest place to swim. This is often near the bank or shore. Look up and around frequently. Wear a brightly coloured swim cap. Use a tow float. If you can, persuade a friend or family member to kayak or SUP next to you. Swim in a group. Carry a whistle so you can attract attention if necessary.

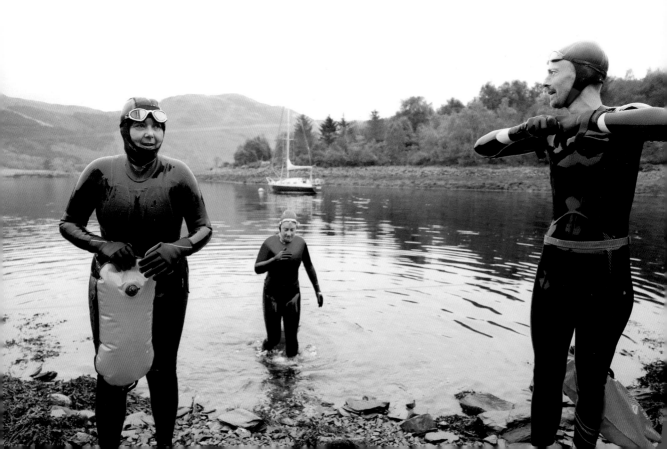

OTHER CREATURES THAT MIGHT HURT YOU

Unlike in swimming pools, we share natural water with other animals, some of which can threaten your physical safety, so a degree of caution is only prudent.

Freshwater Creatures

In the UK, rivers and lakes generally don't harbour things that will bite or sting. However, a friend of mine was once bitten on the hand by a pike. We think it was attracted by light reflecting off his watch, so take care if you're wearing flashing silver objects.

However, when swimming in different countries, always check as not all waters are as swimmer friendly. For example, when Martin Strel swam the length of the Amazon, he had to worry about piranha, crocodiles and bull sharks, among other things. Wing Commander Paramvir Singh reported encountering venomous river snakes and a fearsome gharial (a type of freshwater crocodile) while swimming the length of the Ganges.

Sea Creatures

The sea is also home to creatures that might harm you. For example, sea urchins are common and can cause puncture wounds with their spines. In some cases, the spines are venomous and may sting, or they can become lodged in the skin causing infection. I know one swimmer who developed a nasty (but fortunately temporary) rash after an encounter with a sea cucumber. In the warm coastal waters of the Pacific or Indian Ocean, you may encounter highly venomous sea snakes. However, bites and reported human fatalities are extremely rare. My general rule for anything I'm unsure of in the sea is to observe it from a safe distance and leave it alone.

Sharks, while widely feared, only attack a handful of people each year. On the other hand, humans kill sharks in their thousands. They have more cause to be frightened of us than we of them. Shark attacks are more likely in some parts of the world than others. They're rare enough that sometimes shark attacks on the other side of the planet make global news. If you're swimming anywhere that is visited by sharks, pay attention to what the locals do and the times they swim. There are wetsuits now that are supposed to have anti-shark patterns or, on some long-distance swims where sharks are known to be present, swimmers sometimes use electronic shark repellents.

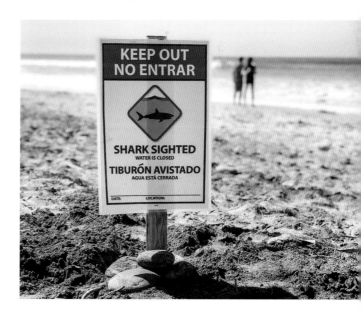

There are hundreds of species of jellyfish around the world, as well as other organisms such as the Portuguese man o' war, that can sting you, some worse than others. Before swimming anywhere new, it's always worth checking with locals. Find out what species of jellyfish are present or if weather conditions might cause them to accumulate anywhere.

It's not just while swimming that you need to be careful. Take care on the beach, too. Weever fish are common around UK, European and North African beaches and deliver a nasty sting if you're unlucky enough to stand on one. They can survive for a time out of water and sometimes lie buried in the sand when the tide has gone out. You can reduce the risk of a sting by wearing beach shoes or neoprene socks. The treatment for a sting is to soak your foot in hot water.

In Florida and many other parts of the world stingrays sometimes bury themselves in shallow water close to the shore. To avoid standing on one, do the stingray shuffle. Shuffling causes vibrations that the stingrays detect, giving them a chance to move away.

Think First

We've looked at lots of hazards in natural waters and I've shared a couple of examples of when things have gone wrong on my swims. This isn't meant to alarm you or put you off, rather to provide the information you need to swim safely. I've had hundreds of amazing outdoor swims during which only good things have happened and very few with adverse outcomes – and those could have been avoided. The best safety advice I can give is to think before you swim and ask local swimmers if there is anything you're unsure about.

How to treat a jellyfish sting

The first aid treatment for a jellyfish sting is to wash the sting with seawater (not fresh water, or urine, which is a popular myth). If there are any visible spines, carefully remove them with tweezers or the edge of a credit card. If possible, soak the area with hot water (or apply hot, wet flannels) for 30 minutes. You can take over-the-counter painkillers if desired. Seek medical assistance if there is any sign of breathing difficulties or severe allergic reaction.

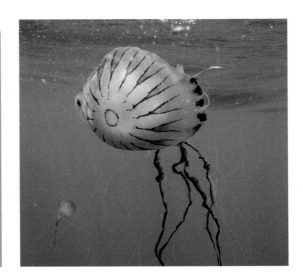

Every now and then, someone forwards me a story about a great white heading for the coast of England. It's usually some fisherman's tale that's recycled periodically when newspapers are running short of real news to write about. It's plausible, given that all our oceans are connected, and, Jaws' casts a long shadow. Unlikely as it is, I still get heart-in-mouth moments in the sea and I know many other swimmers do too. It only takes a shadow made by a cloud passing in front of the sun or a piece of seaweed brushing against my leg to cause my pulse to quicken.

My worst, Jaws' moment in the UK came while swimming off a quiet beach in north Cornwall. I'd swum quite far out to play in the waves when something popped up next to me. I'm short-sighted and didn't see clearly, but it looked big. I raced back to shore and sprinted on to the beach. Once I'd calmed down and put my glasses on, I saw it was a seal and my panic was wasted. Still, I didn't go back in the water that day.

I don't know any cure for fear of sharks except to swim in the sea more often. I've found that the more encounters I've had with things that aren't sharks, the safer I feel. I sometimes suggest swimming with someone slower – it's a joke, but still...

As for jellyfish, they terrified me for years. Long-distance swimmer Adam Walker once showed me a picture of the all-over body burns he collected from jellyfish while swimming the Molokai Channel in Hawaii. Adam still managed to complete that swim, despite near paralysing pain. I know swimmers who have had to terminate swims because of jellyfish stings. However, these are examples of extraordinary swimmers taking on the world's toughest swims.

I lost my extreme fear of jellyfish after being stung by a mauve stinger in Italy. I was in a race and felt a sharp sting in my shoulder and electrical tingles down my arm. I didn't see the culprit, but I felt it roll across my back, stinging me again two or three more times. It was nasty, perhaps on par with a wasp sting, maybe a little worse. I certainly wouldn't seek out being stung again, but somehow knowing what it's like lessens the fear.

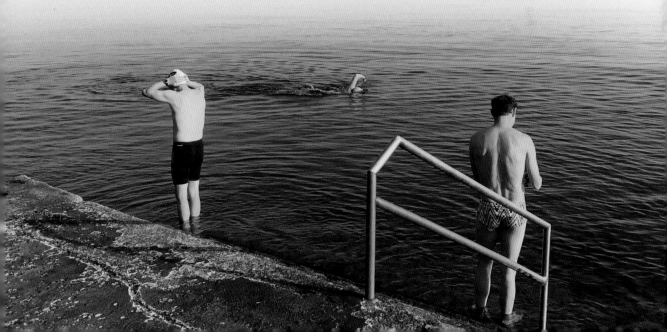

SWIMMING WHATEVER THE WEATHER (ALMOST)

Swimmers will venture into the water in a wide range of weather conditions. Sometimes, the more extreme the conditions, the more people want to swim. On one WhatsApp swimming group I'm a member of, the greatest excitement last year was the prospect of swimming in the snow. It's part of the appeal of swimming in nature. But weather conditions add new risks to swimming that you need to be aware of. Some are obvious, some less so.

Sunshine and Hot Weather

Hot weather and sunshine should provide ideal outdoor swimming conditions, and mostly they do, but take care not to get sunburnt, which is surprisingly easy when swimming. Second, water warms up much more slowly than the air, so on hot days the water temperature will often be significantly lower than the air temperature. Cold water shock is therefore still a risk. Also note that the surface layer of water is often warm, while deeper water is cool.

A prolonged dry spell can promote algae growth that may be detrimental to water quality. Blue-green algae in particular is toxic (*see* p. 39). If the water is covered in a dense, green, paint-like layer, do not swim. Finally, hot weather can be a precursor to storms.

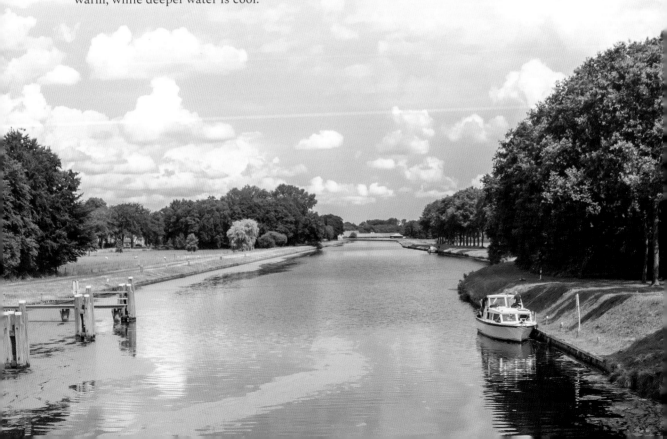

Electrical Storms

You should avoid swimming in electrical storms. If you're swimming and you see lightning or hear thunder, you should leave the water and seek safe shelter in a building or a car. Lightning tends to strike the tallest local object. When you're swimming, that is likely to be any part of your body that's out of the water. Also, water conducts electricity, so even if you're not hit directly, you could still be electrocuted by a nearby strike.

Only get on to a boat if it will get you to shore and safe shelter quicker than swimming. Being on a boat is possibly more dangerous than being in the water. And definitely don't stand on the beach, dripping wet, watching the storm roll through.

Rain

Many swimmers love swimming in the rain. It creates a special atmosphere on the water, especially those gentle rain showers that happen with no wind. The water goes completely flat and is punctured by the raindrops. I recommend watching the rain with your eyes at water level, listening to its patter, deeply inhaling its scent and fully savouring the moment with all your senses.

There are, however, some practical considerations. Try to keep your clothes dry as you will need them so you can warm up after swimming. Take extra care getting into and out of the water as banks and rocks could be more slippery than usual. You also need to be aware that heavy or prolonged rain can adversely affect water quality and conditions.

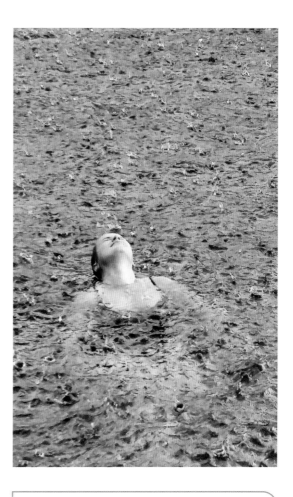

When it rains

- Water running off the land may be contaminated.
- Heavy rain can cause sewage to spill into rivers or the sea. Stay away from any pipes discharging into the water.
- Flow and depth in rivers can change suddenly due to rain.

Fog

Some of my most beautiful swims have been early in the morning with thick mist lying across the water. But swimming in fog has obvious risks. Always use a tow float for additional visibility and consider putting a light inside it. Stay within sight of your exit point and pay extra attention to your surroundings. Don't swim in thick fog.

Snow and Ice

Snow is rare where I live, but the last time it happened, while our neighbours wrapped up in winter coats to build snowmen, I put on my swimming trunks and dashed to the river. I wasn't alone. The chance to swim in the snow created a buzz in my local swimming group, as I'm sure it did in many others.

Swimming in the snow requires the same precautions as any cold water dip. Be careful not to get carried away by the excitement and stay in too long. If roads are blocked or icy, it might take emergency vehicles longer to reach you. Pay attention to your entry and exit points as they may be slippery, and ensure you pack your clothes securely so they stay dry and you can dress quickly afterwards.

You may have seen pictures of swimmers breaking the ice to dip, but I don't recommend this for beginners. However, should you want to try it, watch out for sharp edges on the ice and consider wearing gloves to protect your hands. Do not linger in the water.

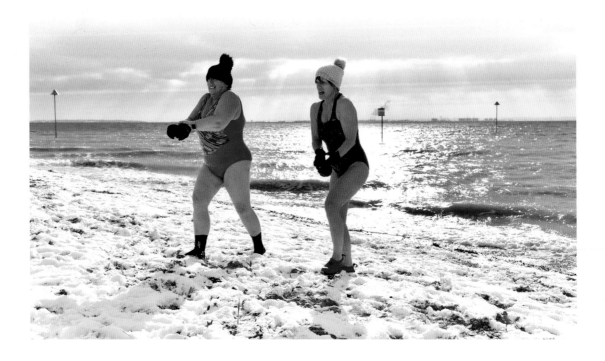

Wind

Wind can make a swim exhilarating, but it can add complications. Most obviously, wind roughens up the water surface, and that can play havoc with your swimming stroke and breathing. Larger inland bodies of water can develop surprisingly big waves. Conditions can get particularly messy when the wind blows against the current, say in a river or on the sea.

You therefore need to use judgement when deciding whether or not to swim in windy conditions, especially in the sea, which can become treacherous. If you have someone supporting you on a kayak or SUP, you might be able to swim in stronger winds than they can paddle, so keep that in mind when deciding what the limit is.

Remember that wind chill will cool you down faster than usual. Make your swim shorter, and dress quickly and warmly afterwards. Inland waters often collect debris in the wind. Watch out for sticks and branches in the water.

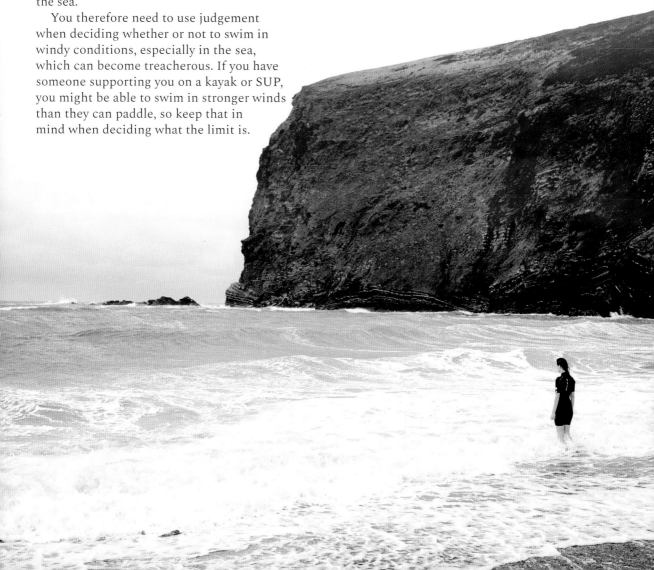

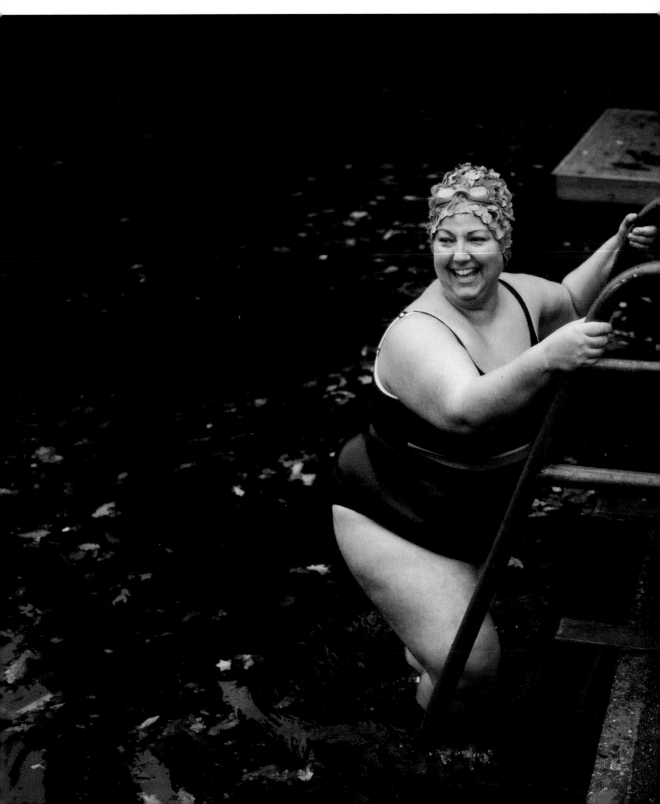

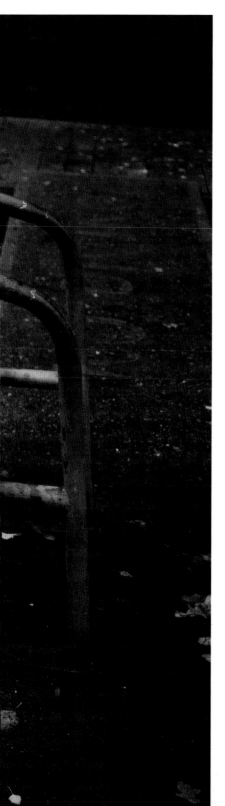

CHAPTER 3

TAKE A SWIM ON THE WILD SIDE

Now you know how to stay safe in and around the water, it's time to start exploring. In this chapter, find out how to discover places for wild swimming, what to do if you prefer to swim with a guide and how to make sure your wild swimming spot stays wild.

WHAT IS WILD SWIMMING?

Much as I enjoy swimming at supervised venues, I love to break away from the circuits and find out what else there is to explore. And there's lots, from tiny pools left behind by the receding tide at the sea and streams that occasionally open up enough for a brief dip, to great rivers, and stunning lakes and lochs.

I think of wild swimming as swimming that isn't controlled, supervised or regulated. Wild swimming feels liberating and slightly eccentric. There are no rules and there is no pressure. You can stretch the definitions of both wild and swimming to their limits.

Swimmers tend to immerse themselves in nature, but you occasionally find wild swimming spots in urban environments, too. The other thing I like about it is that it's usually free.

While hiking, I once stumbled upon a tranquil hidden pool below a spring. The sun, sinking behind the cliffs, had left the rocks around the pool radiating warmth. I stripped and slid into the water, which was breathtakingly cold, but it would be a stretch to call it wild. I swam only in the sense that I took my feet off the bottom for a few seconds and relieved them momentarily from the dull ache of a long day's walking. It was soothing and rejuvenating, but barely a swim. After just a couple of minutes in the water, I spread myself over the heated rocks to dry.

However, I also love swimming in surf and moving water. In winter, with a small group of friends, we sometimes launch ourselves into a murky, swirling river and let the current sweep us downstream, much faster than any of us could swim. That's wild. And fun. But remember, moving water can be dangerous, so don't try anything like this until you have some experience. We plan it carefully, plotting where we will get out and what we'd do if we wanted to exit early or overshoot our planned finish. We discuss the hazards and how we can minimise the risks.

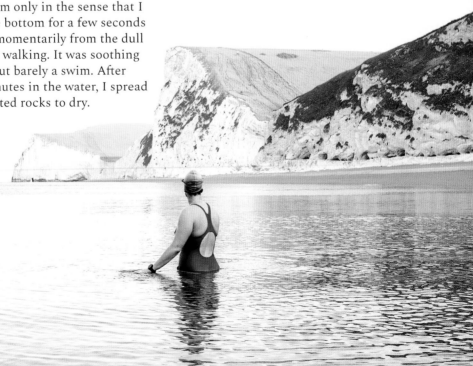

WHERE TO SWIM WILD

There are practical, logistical and sometimes legal challenges in finding wild swimming spots, but it's worth the effort.

On a trip to France once, I asked a local for advice about where to swim. He told me to look for the 'baignade interdite' sign. I followed a winding footpath alongside a stream until I found a spot where it opened up into some beautiful limestone pools, along with the promised sign forbidding bathing, and a few dozen French families picnicking and swimming.

Unlike some places in France, 'No swimming' signs in the UK tend to be taken seriously and I wouldn't advise swimming where they are displayed. Sometimes they are there for good reason and sometimes not, but it's not always obvious which it is. Also England doesn't (yet) have the same widespread cultural acceptance of using our rivers and lakes for family recreation and swimming, although the mood is changing. France, for example, has more than 1000 inland designated bathing spots in lakes and rivers. England has one river and a handful of lakes.

Still, the UK does have plenty of beautiful swimming spots. The fact they are not designated bathing waters does not mean they are not suitable for swimming. The best way to find them is often through one of the many wild swimming guidebooks (*see* Further reading and references on pp. 202–203 for some recommendations). Get one and plan trips around the spots that take your fancy.

You can also find recommendations online. A search for 'best places to swim near...' often turns up some good suggestions.

To find something more personalised, grab an Ordnance Survey map and look for public footpaths that run alongside rivers and other bodies of water. In general, in England, swimming is allowed in navigable rivers, but you could be trespassing if you cross private land to reach the water, hence the need to use public footpaths. Scotland has the right to roam written into law, which (among other things) allows everyone access to inland water for swimming. Always check local laws. In some countries, such as Germany and Sweden, recommended swimming spots are sometimes marked on maps and signposted, but not everywhere is as welcoming.

Finding swim spots with a map adds complications that you need to be aware of. Recommendations from books tend to be spots where people already swim and there is shared knowledge about the best entry points, water quality and any hazards. When you seek out your own spots, you have to discover this for yourself. It's part of the fun, but it adds to the risk. Take your time assessing any new swimming spot and if you are unsure or worried about anything, don't swim.

WILD SWIMMING WHILE TRAVELLING

Almost any trip can be enhanced with a swim – even better if it's a wild swim.

In the late 1980s, I hitch-hiked to Istanbul. While passing through Germany I was given a lift by a man from Berlin in a rental van. It turns out that he'd stolen the van and was planning to drive to southern Europe to sell it, but that's another story. After several hours of driving in the heat, he suddenly pulled off the road and announced he was going for a swim. He'd glimpsed a river running parallel to the road. While I searched my backpack for my trunks and a towel, he'd already stripped (completely) and plunged into the water. He thought it hilarious and odd that I wanted to wear a costume and explained it was normal to swim naked in rivers in Germany.

I've travelled in Germany many times since then. While nudity may not be so prevalent as Man-in-a-Stolen-Van suggested, it definitely exists. More importantly, as in France, swimming in lakes and rivers is more normal than in England, with inland bathing spots signposted or marked on maps, and information about water quality provided.

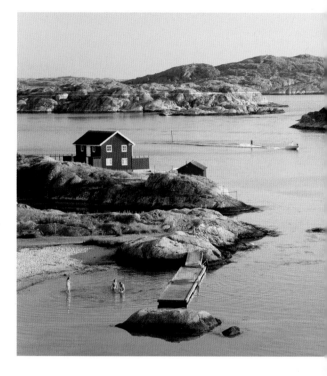

Every country has its own relationship with swimming and water. In some ways, the UK is unusually restricted and nervous. The phrase 'wild swimming' in part embodies a spirit of rebellion and non-conformity that's required in the UK and that isn't needed elsewhere. Adding swimming to the list of things you might do when you visit another country gives you another lens through which to see a different culture. It's worth carrying a costume wherever you go for that experience, but do take care to respect local laws, traditions and customs.

Driving through Sweden one summer, Google diverted us from our expected road along the coast on to an inland road, telling us we were on the 'best route'. While we were debating the criteria Google might have used to determine 'best', we rounded a corner and saw a long, narrow lake sparkling in the afternoon sun. After that, we spotted a sign for a bathing spot next to an unmade road, so naturally we turned off to have a look. Google clearly knows what's best for me as the track opened up into a stunning but deserted swimming spot. Over the course of several days, we stumbled across multiple lakes with signposted swimming spots and a relaxed, no-fuss approach to swimming in them.

CONNECT WITH A LOCAL SWIM GROUP

Perhaps the safest and most enjoyable way to start wild swimming is to connect with an existing swimming group.

There are outdoor swimming groups all around the world. Some of these are formal bodies with a constitution and paid membership. Formalisation brings benefits, such as public liability insurance for swim group leaders and possible negotiation clout with access to swim spots.

The majority, however, are informal, connecting through social media. Some have regular meeting spots and times. Others are more ad hoc. I'm a member of several on WhatsApp and Facebook, with the Facebook ones tending to be more open to random swimmers joining. Search for 'outdoor swimmers' and see what pops up.

Or you could find a local group of 'Bluetits', part of a growing international network of outdoor swimming groups. Sian Richardson started the Bluetits in September 2014 in Pembrokeshire, Wales, when she decided to swim in the sea through the winter. She was soon joined by others and within seven years, there were more than 15,000 Bluetits around the world.

Swimming groups are usually welcoming and friendly, and know the best local spots to swim. However, rather than just asking on social media for advice on where to swim, join the group on one of its regular swims. Get to know the swimmers. Learn from their experience and share yours. And if you don't yet have any swimming experiences, share food instead.

Groups aren't for everyone and there is no requirement to join one. But, if you do, make sure you familiarise yourself with any guidelines. These typically state that swimmers must take responsibility for their own safety and cannot hold the volunteer swim organisers liable for any harm that might come to them while swimming.

Keep your wild swim spot wild

My personal favourite wild swim spots are those that are the least spoiled. I hate finding litter, either on the bank or in the water. It upsets me to see plants callously trampled over. Outdoor swimmers, in my experience, are good custodians of nature and respectful of the environments they swim in. But sometimes we forget or get clumsy. Please try to do the following:

- Take away all your own litter and any other litter you can find.
- Take care not to damage plants or disturb wildlife, especially when entering and exiting the water.
- Avoid putting on sunscreen immediately before swimming as it washes off and pollutes the water.
- If you need to wear sunscreen while swimming, choose an eco-friendly reef-safe brand.
- Help prevent the spread of invasive species. Always wash and fully dry your wetsuit between swims in different locations.

GUIDED WILD SWIMS

Rather than joining an informal group swim, another option worth exploring is to join a guided swim. Increasing numbers of swimmers are taking coaching and lifeguarding qualifications, and setting themselves up in business as swimming guides around their local areas.

Swimming guides are great, because they will usually know the most beautiful spots, the best times to go and the easiest ways to get in and out of the water.

While you have to pay for guided swims, rather than swimming free with a group or finding your own spot, you have the reassurance that a qualified guide is fully insured to take people swimming and will have done detailed risk assessments. Try searching for 'wild swim guides in ...' or 'outdoor swimming guides near ...' and see if anyone pops up. Also *see* Further reading and references on pp. 102–103 for some recommendations.

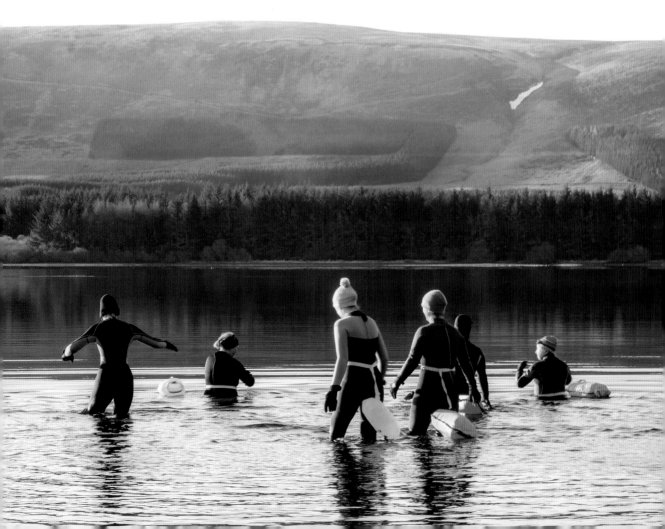

SWIMMING IN THE SEA

Although I grew up and still live far from the coast, the sea has a magical appeal. I assume this comes from my mother, who grew up in Devon and, when she had the opportunity, moved to Cornwall partly to be near the sea. I therefore had the good fortune to spend many holidays exploring the north Cornish coast and swimming in the Atlantic.

The sea feels different to fresh water. Because of the salt, you are more buoyant, making it easier to float. I think – and I'm not alone in this – that salt water seems warmer than fresh water for the same objective temperature measurement. It also feels softer on my skin, although that's misleading as you're more likely to suffer chafing in salt water than fresh.

Oceans hold many delights for wild swimmers, from waves for playing in or surfing on, to iconic long-distance swimming challenges. It also hides many dangers.

Quick tips for sea swimming

- Beach shoes or neoprene socks can greatly ease your entry and exit to the sea over pebbles or sharp rocks, and protect your feet from weever fish, stingrays and sharp objects.
- Goggles can be easily knocked off in surf. If you're playing in the waves, either go without or consider putting them under a swimming cap to keep them in place.
- Duck under incoming waves to swim out into calmer water.
- Ride the waves coming back into shore, but beware of underwater objects.
- Keep an eye on a fixed point on shore to make sure you're not drifting.
- Relax when you're swimming in rough water and enjoy the power of the sea.

The obvious place to start swimming in the sea is a lifeguarded beach where you know safety cover is in place. The trouble is, these places are often the most popular and crowded. It's hard to enjoy a swim if you're constantly worried about being struck by a surfer. Luckily, in many places, it doesn't take a lot of effort to find quieter spots. The trick, often, is to scour the map for beaches that are a mile or two from the nearest car park and accessible only by footpath.

Alternatively, look for guides to hidden beaches (which seems somewhat ironic to me) or try a quick internet search. 'Quiet beach near …' occasionally turns up a pleasant surprise. But please remember, you need to do your own risk assessment at secluded beaches. You may be far from help if you need it and your phone might not work. Make sure you familiarise yourself with the safety guidance in Chapter 2 and check out the tips for swimming in waves and rough water in Chapter 9.

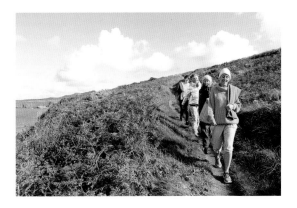

WILD SWIMMING IN THE DARK

Water has a different allure at night and wild swimming in the dark can be a wonderful experience. Full moon swimming, is a 'thing'. The reduced visibility and the late or early hour add a dose of trepidation and excitement. It does also add to the risks, so you do need to think about what you're doing. It's best to wait until you've done a few swims in daylight before trying this out.

It's a good idea to make yourself highly visible for a night swim. One trick is to put a bright torch inside your tow float, which turns it into a lovely glow-in-the-dark safety device. Alternatively, clip a waterproof safety light to the back of your goggles. Some swimmers use glow-sticks but I'm not a fan as they are not recyclable.

Air cools down faster than water in the night. Often, the water temperature at night is almost identical to what it was during the day, while outside is much cooler. This can make getting into the water a pleasant surprise. However, you may find it takes longer to warm up again after your swim. Bring plenty of warm layers, a warm drink and a snack for after. Plan how you will find your clothes and dress in the dark. Arrange them so you can put them on as quickly as possible.

On a university canoeing trip to the South of France, one night I was so tempted by the moon's glitter path across the surf that I spontaneously stripped on the beach and went in for a swim. My fellow travellers, being students, thought it was a good idea to hide my clothes. Luckily it was a warm night and I didn't freeze, but if you are tempted by a moonlit skinny dip, it's probably best to make sure nobody is going to move your stuff.

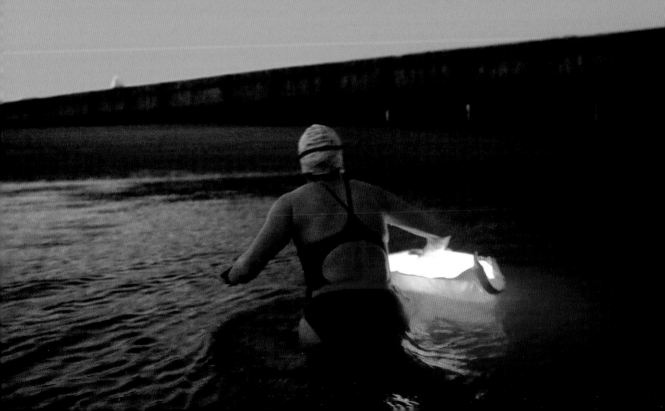

ACCESS RIGHTS

In much of the world there is no inalienable right to swim. Whether you can swim or not is defined by a mixture of law and tradition or may not be specified one way or the other. The land around or adjacent to water may be privately owned, which can stop you even reaching it.

In some instances, the right to swim in water on public land is removed or restricted by local authorities, for a range of reasons, including real and imagined dangers. Wherever you want to swim, it's best to seek local opinion.

Access to much of the swimmable inland water in England and Wales is, sadly, contested or illegal. Even the government doesn't always know. A government webpage about the River Wye says:

- There is no confirmed legal right of navigation upstream of Hay Bridge.
- Access to navigate the upper Wye is disputed.

If you are in Scotland, the situation is better due to the right to roam laws.

British Canoeing, the national governing body for canoeing, says there is 70,671km (43,913 miles) of inland water resource in England and Wales, but that less than 4 per cent of rivers have a clear right of access. Water that is suitable for paddling is often also suitable for swimming, and paddlers and swimmers have similar access rights.

As mentioned previously, you do have a legal right to swim in most navigable rivers in England and Wales – 'navigable' in the legal rather than practical sense.

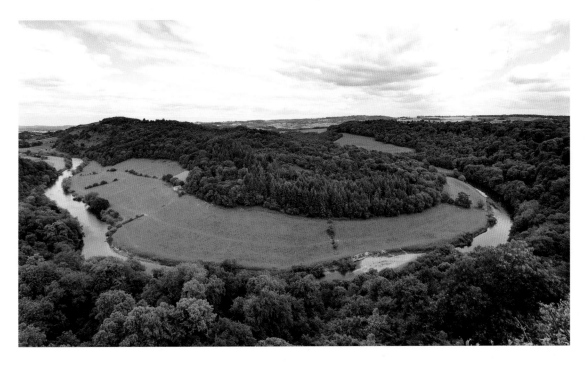

However, swimming in navigable rivers is all well and good, but they are the main roads of our waterways and have a major downside of often being busy with boat traffic. More relaxed swimming spots tend to be found on

You can find a map of navigable rivers on the Canal & River Trust website. The trust says there are 435km (270 miles) of such water in England and Wales.

smaller rivers and streams. If you can access these from public land or footpaths, there is a strong argument for being allowed to swim there. There are also places where people have traditionally swum and where swimming is accepted. Local knowledge is most useful in these circumstances. Note, mostly, swimming in canals is neither allowed nor desirable.

Many parts of Britain, such as the M4 corridor and the area around Cirencester, are rich in lakes created from old quarries and gravel pits. While some abandoned quarries are dangerous to swim in, many are ideal, with

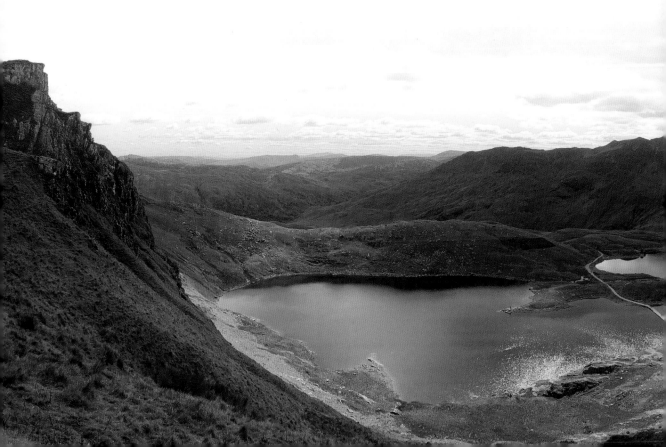

clear, good-quality water. However, as these are mostly on private land, you can't swim there, except for those that offer commercial supervised swimming. On the other hand, you can swim in most of the lakes in the Lake District and Snowdonia National Park. You will have to check other lakes and ponds you come across on a case-by-case basis. If they are on private land, or you need to cross private land to reach the water, you should ask the landowner's permission.

Reservoirs are a different matter. Mostly these are owned and looked after by privatised water companies, who have a legal duty to offer recreational access to the water and surrounding land. While you often see other watersports in action, swimming is usually forbidden. The water companies typically say this is for safety reasons – and it's true that you wouldn't want to swim near a spillway or any machinery – but many reservoirs have the potential to offer safe swimming. Hopefully, they will do so in the future.

Ending on a positive note, swimmers in the UK do have free and undisputed access to the sea – something that isn't a global right.

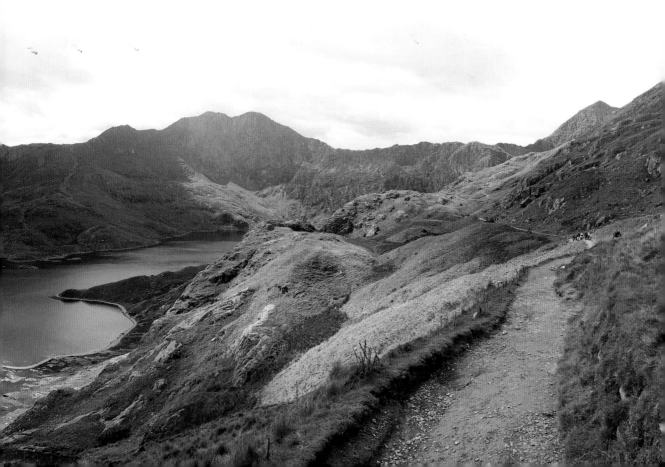

CASE STUDY
HELPING MARGINALISED GROUPS ACCESS OUTDOOR SWIMMING

Maggy Blagrove, director and founder of Open Minds Active, works with marginalised groups and helps introduce people to outdoor swimming. Here she describes some of the barriers they face.

Geography, history and culture mean access to outdoor swimming is unequal. But why shouldn't anyone be able to enjoy its benefits? They can, but sometimes they need help from organisations like Open Minds Active, a social impact organisation that works to break down barriers and promote wild swimming to groups who might not normally access green or blue spaces ('blue' meaning water).

The first barrier is a lack of awareness. If outdoor swimming is not promoted within specific communities, they won't know it exists, or they just assume it's not for them. To tackle this, we talk to groups about the benefits of open water swimming, and build links between clubs and coaches at venues that communities can access.

A second issue is a lack of transport. For those living in inner cities, access to open water can be a challenge. Generally wild swim spots are not on bus routes. Even for drivers, there is a fear of getting lost. Open Minds Active operates a car share scheme and volunteers take small groups so they can learn the routes and work out how to get there independently in future.

Many of the adult women of colour that Open Minds Active work with lack confidence around open water and find the concept terrifying. There is a real fear among some ethnic minorities that open water is cold, dangerous and dirty. Many women of colour lack the swim skills to swim in a pool, let alone outdoors. This, coupled with a lack of representation in swimming at both elite and community level, fosters an assumption that it's not for them. To counteract this, we run initiatives led by representatives from marginalised communities who inspire local women to learn to swim in a pool and then progress to open water as their skills and confidence improves.

One of these representatives is Wafa Suliman, a former professional swimmer in her home country of Sudan. She manages the Open Minds Active learn to swim programme and, as a Muslim woman, helps break down many of the cultural and practical barriers to swimming as well as dispel many of the stereotypes and myths. As a result, increasing numbers of women from marginalised groups in Bristol are discovering the joys of outdoor swimming.

Wafa Suliman's top tips for getting started in outdoor swimming

1. For many women of colour, hair can be a big issue and so finding the right swim cap is key. We use Soul Caps for the women in our sessions as they come in a range of sizes to suit all kinds of volume. This is a real game changer for many women as they love the look and feel of the caps, and feel reassured that their hair is protected against the elements.

2. Wetsuits can be a minefield to choose but also incredibly helpful, especially around cultural sensitivities. The Muslim women we work with like that they are fully covered when swimming, and that the wetsuits provide extra buoyancy and warmth.

3. A basic changing towel is also great as this protects modesty when there are no changing facilities and doesn't have to cost a fortune.

4. A good-sized bag for wet kit is a must. Again, it doesn't have to be flashy or expensive – a bag-for-life or strong fabric bag work really well.

5. Tow floats are a must as they provide visibility. They are not a lifesaving device, but do give novice swimmers confidence in open water. The women in our sessions love them as they hold on to them while they float on their backs or their fronts for a rest and a chat.

6. Make sure swimming skills are at a good level in a pool environment before venturing outside. Contact an open water coach or local club in your area to do an introduction session. They will show you all the best spots and teach you valuable acclimatisation and open water skills. Never try open water swimming alone.

7. Ideally, start open water swimming in the summer months when the water temperatures are warmer and then you can steadily acclimatise as the weather gets cooler. Know your limits and don't stay in too long.

8. Every part of the country has its wild swim spots to explore, but always go with an experienced swimmer or coach who knows the area, and always look out for each other.

Open Minds Active runs introduction sessions in the summer months in Bristol specifically for women of colour, but there are always other groups popping up on Facebook or other organisations across the country that are starting to do the same.

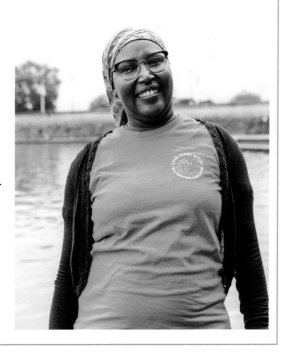

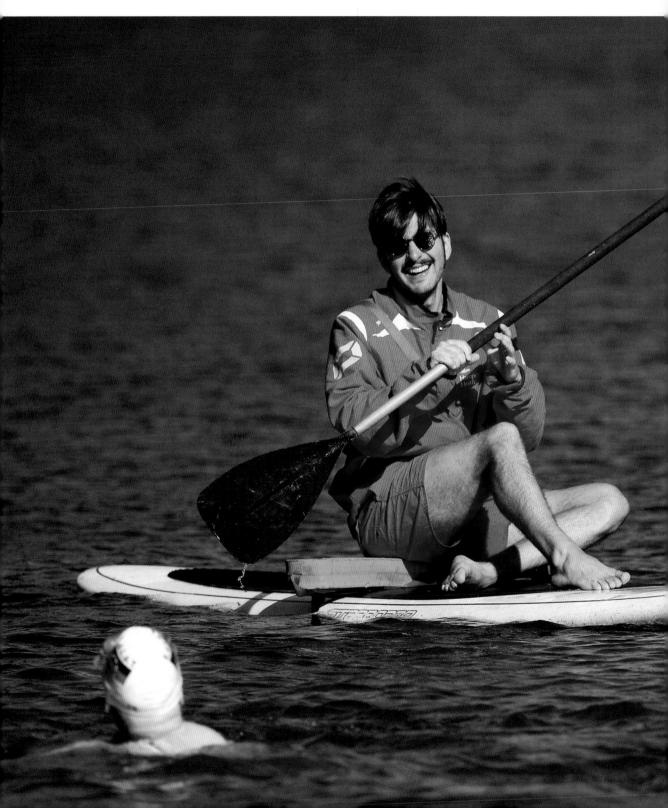

CHAPTER 4

SWIMMING AT SUPERVISED VENUES

Supervised outdoor swimming venues offer safe, water-quality tested, lifeguarded open water swimming, often with measured distances. Many also offer coaching services, making them ideal for beginners and for swim training.

WHAT ARE OPEN WATER SWIMMING VENUES?

If you're looking for somewhere safe and life-guarded to swim outdoors, see if you can find a supervised venue.

Supervised swimming venues are a relatively new phenomenon. I remember, in the 1970s, my mother taking us to a gravel pit lake for swimming, but we just messed about in the water, like you do at a seaside beach. I don't recall any lifeguards or any payment to get in and neither does my mother. Nor were there any measured swimming loops or designated swimming areas. Now, those same gravel pits have become part of the Cotswold Water Park.

Many of the lakes in the park offer water-based activities such as windsurfing, kayaking and fishing. A growing number allow swimming, but differently to how it was when I was growing up. There are now designated swim areas and training loops, swim sessions are lifeguarded and coaches provide courses for beginners through to competitive swimmers. And you have to pay for access.

In the UK, supervised venues started appearing in the 1990s as a place for triathletes to train. The first triathlon in the UK took place in 1983 and the sport grew rapidly through the 1990s and 2000s. Enterprising coaches spotted an opportunity and set up swim courses in lakes, modelled on those you see in triathlon.

Triathlon coach Rick Kiddle set up one of the first open water swimming venues at Heron Lake. He says: 'We were probably the first to really run a venue to its potential. We marketed it and ran it commercially with safety, coaching, equipment sales and hire as well as a good offering of drink and food.'

The set-up today of many supervised venues still reflects this. However, the clientele has changed over the years. Triathletes still do their timed circuits, but they've been joined and often outnumbered by swimmers who have no interest in triathlon. Rick, who now runs the National Open Water Coaches Association (NOWCA), says in the beginning they had around 90 per cent triathletes and 10 per cent swimmers. Now it is more like 80 per cent swimmers and 20 per cent triathletes. Swimmer numbers were boosted during 2020's lockdown with an influx of displaced pool swimmers who continued swimming outside after pools reopened. There are more than 100 supervised outdoor swimming venues across the UK.

Key benefits of supervised venues

- Safety cover provided by qualified lifeguards.
- Water quality regularly checked.
- You can swim alone.
- Measured distances for training.
- Many have changing and shower facilities.

Lifeguards and Water Testing

Venues offer something for swimmers at almost any level. I tend to head to one when I want to do a long, uninterrupted swim. You can put your head down and get on with swimming without worrying about boats or other water users, and be confident that the water quality has been tested and meets bathing water standards.

I also like the reassurance that supervised venues are watched over by lifeguards, who should either hold a National Vocational Beach Lifeguard Qualification (NVBLQ) or an Open Water Lifeguard (OWL) qualification.

Each venue organises safety cover differently with lifeguards either on the water in kayaks or on SUPS, or watching from shore. Many have both. I try to make a point of mentally noting where the lifeguards are when I swim, just in case I need to attract their attention for any reason.

Because of the safety measures in place, supervised venues are one of the few places I'm comfortable swimming alone. However, there is always a good chance I will meet someone I know when I go, which brings me to my next point: community.

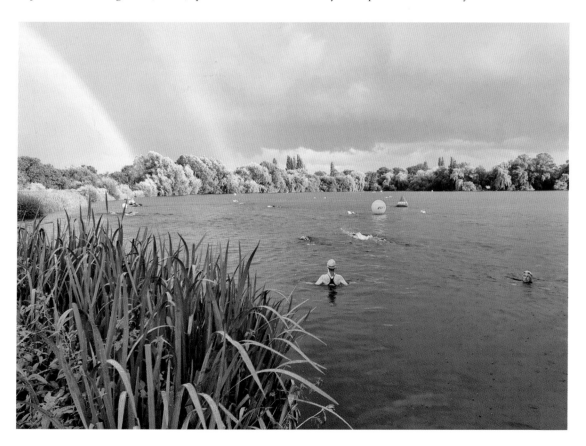

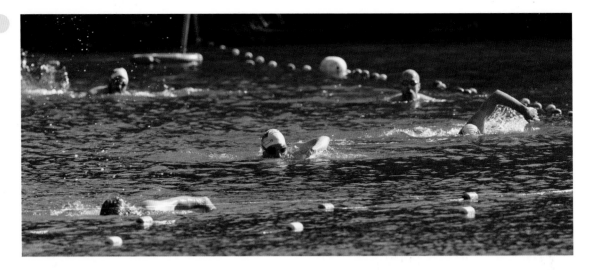

Community

The best venues (in my opinion) foster a strong sense of community. Some rely on volunteers to help provide safety cover and assist with administration, which builds a community feeling. This often becomes more pronounced during the colder months of the year when fewer people swim. Sometimes the numbers don't stack up for commercial operation, but by supporting volunteering, they can continue offering swims.

Venues may also host low-key races, social events or invite retailers to exhibit. This may, for example, give swimmers the chance to try wetsuits before committing to buy.

Limited Opening Hours

At a lot of venues, the water is shared with other users. Many were originally waterskiing or wakeboarding lakes and still operate as such. Obviously, you can't have swimmers and waterskiers using the water at the same time and, as the waterskiers were often there first, swimmers tend to get the early morning and late evening slots.

Even lakes that don't have those restrictions tend to offer similar opening times. It seems swimmers like to swim at sunrise and sunset anyway. During working hours, there often isn't sufficient demand for lakes to offer swimming commercially.

Always check a venue's opening hours and booking requirements before turning up. Visit their website in advance of swimming and download their booking app and disclaimer forms if required.

What to Expect on Your First Visit

Getting started in outdoor swimming can be intimidating. Going to a supervised venue where there will be lots of more experienced swimmers, perhaps even more so. However, most venues do a brilliant job of welcoming and looking after new swimmers. Some run specific induction sessions for beginners. At others there are qualified outdoor swimming coaches who can help you get started. It's best to make enquiries before you book.

If you are already a confident swimmer and have some outdoor swimming experience, you may not need these introductory sessions, but don't be surprised if you are asked to demonstrate your swimming competence.

SUPERVISED VENUES - FAQS

Like swimming pools, supervised venues have certain ways of doing things and you might feel a little intimidated or unsure on your first visit and have a few questions. That's normal. Here are some of the most frequently asked:

How will I know a venue is run by a safe operator?

Unlike public swimming pools, venues don't have to follow any particular guidelines. However, they will need to demonstrate to their insurers that they run a safe operation. In addition, venues now have an option to seek accreditation and reassure swimmers of their safety standards through Beyond Swim, a joint initiative between the British Triathlon Federation and Swim England (the national governing bodies for triathlon and swimming) and the Royal Life Saving Society UK. Beyond Swim replaces a previous accreditation system known as SH$_2$OUT, which you might still see referenced.

Separately, NOWCA offers venues a booking and swimmer tracking system. With the NOWCA system, swimmers are given a band with a radio-frequency identification (RFID) tag, which they use to check in and out of the water. The band connects to a database that holds swimmers' emergency details.

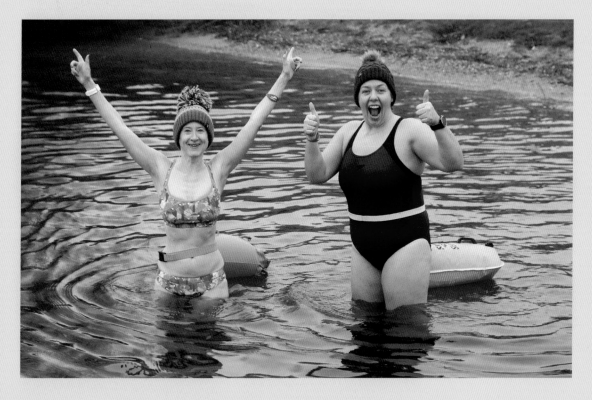

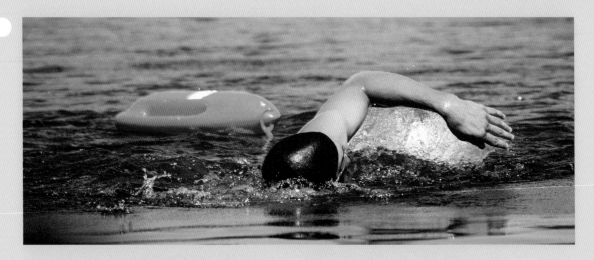

Will I have to swim long-distance circuits?

When venues catered primarily for triathletes, they frequently set up with relatively long loops: 750m or 800m (820 or 875 yards) is common. Increasingly, many now have options for shorter loops of between 200m and 400m (220 and 440 yards). At some, there are areas for swimming where you can stay close to the exit.

While 750m (820 yards) sounds like a long way if you're used to a 25m (27.5-yard) swimming pool (it's equivalent to 30 lengths), you will find you soon enjoy the opportunity to swim without having to turn around at a wall all the time.

A few venues now also provide a 'lido' area, where you can swim as you like.

Do I have to wear a wetsuit?

Venues have their own policies. Some insist all swimmers wear wetsuits at all times. Others have rules that depend on the water temperature. Alternatively, you may be asked to demonstrate your swimming competence and experience before being allowed to swim without a wetsuit. Some allow you to do what you want. Always check first.

Do I have to use a tow float?

Obligatory use of tow floats is becoming increasingly common at venues as it makes it so much easier for lifeguards to keep track of all the swimmers in the water and see where they are at all times. In addition, venue operators find they provide swimmers with reassurance and, if they do get into difficulties, give swimmers something to hold on to until a lifeguard can reach them. I recommend using one even if it's not required, especially if you are swimming without a wetsuit.

How good a swimmer do I need to be?

This depends on the venue. For venues with circuits, I suggest being able to swim continuously for twice the distance of the shortest circuit. Speed, style and technique don't matter as long as you are comfortable and relaxed in the water. While you don't have the option to rest at a wall like you do in a swimming pool, a wetsuit (if you choose to wear one) provides enough buoyancy to keep you afloat without any effort. You should find it easier to swim in one than without. If you're unsure, sign up for an induction section or a series of lessons to help build your confidence.

Will I get swum over by faster swimmers and triathletes?

Hopefully not! While mixing swimmers of different speeds in pools can lead to lane rage, there is plenty of space in lakes for everyone to swim as they like and not interfere with anyone else. Faster swimmers are encouraged to take a wide line and give plenty of space when overtaking.

Can I take my children?

Not always, unfortunately. But some venues welcome youngsters. You will need to check with the venue directly.

What about facilities for swimmers with disabilities?

Again, this is venue dependent and also depends what your needs are. Heron Lake, near Staines, is home to the British Disabled Water Ski and Wakeboard Association. As such, it has facilities for swimmers with disabilities, such as hardstanding parking close to the water and a ramp to enter the water. It also offers open water swimming sessions. The best option is to contact the venue operator. Most will be willing to help where they can.

How do I find a supervised venue?

Check out the venue listings on *Outdoor Swimmer*'s and Swim England's websites. Beyond Swim have a listing of accredited venues.

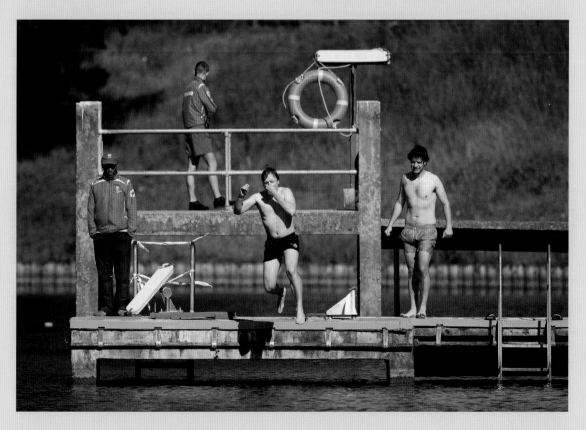

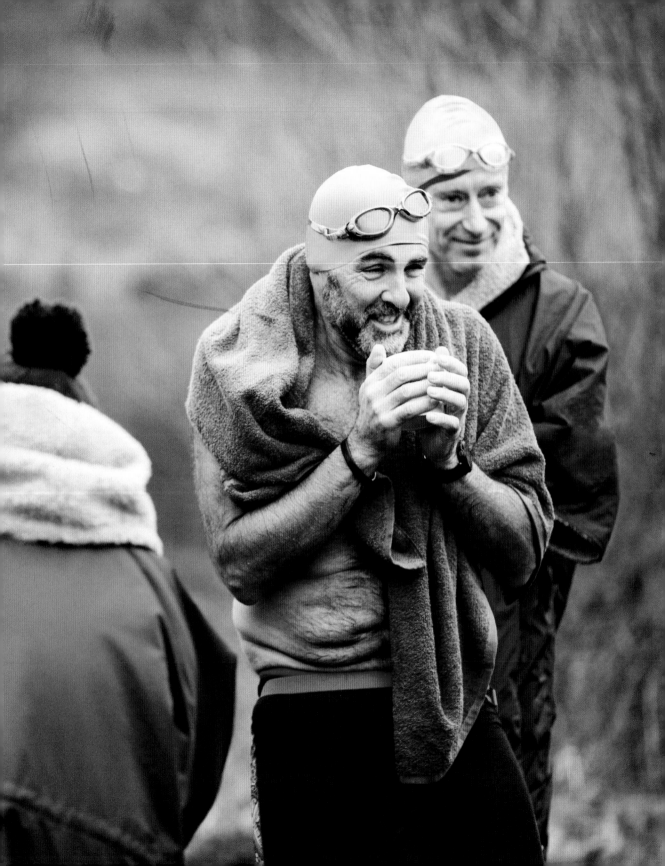

MY STORY

Encouraging men to swim and talk

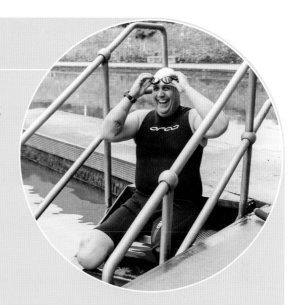

The best thing for me about outdoor swimming is the community. You meet such an amazing range of people in the water. I could be swimming with a lord and a bus driver and you wouldn't know the difference. It's a massive leveller. Then, I think because my injuries are very visible [Simon lost his legs to an improvised explosive device in Afghanistan], a lot of people talk to me and share their own stories about difficult things they are going through and how swimming helps. Outdoor swimming, anecdotally at least, seems to help alleviate multiple problems.

It's quite a female-dominated activity so one of the things I try to do is encourage more men to swim. I know it's a cliché, but men do seem less likely to open up and talk about stuff. Outdoor swimming – especially winter swimming – somehow gives us the space and platform to talk, and I can see it makes a real difference to the people I swim with.

Swimming itself gives me a sense of achievement and well-being, even if some days I just get in the water, float around a bit and chat. I do like to aim for challenges, too. Nothing too big, but enough to push me to
train and keep fit. This year, I'm aiming to swim the length of Ullswater in the Lake District with a friend. We'll probably swim it slower than if I were to do it alone, but that's not the point. I still need to train and get fit for it. I also love swimming with my 10-year-old daughter.*

My advice for anyone who is nervous about outdoor swimming is to lower the barriers and expectations. Go somewhere suitable for beginners with easy entry, no boat traffic or waves, and clear water. Wear a wetsuit so you don't have to worry about the cold. You can always remove it later. Swim at your pace and do as much or as little as you're comfortable with.

SIMON HARMER

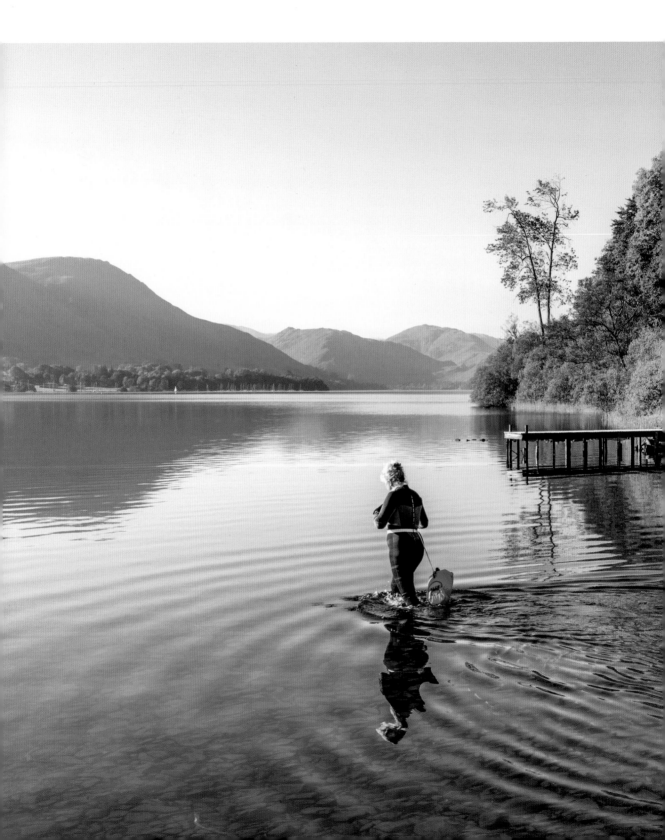

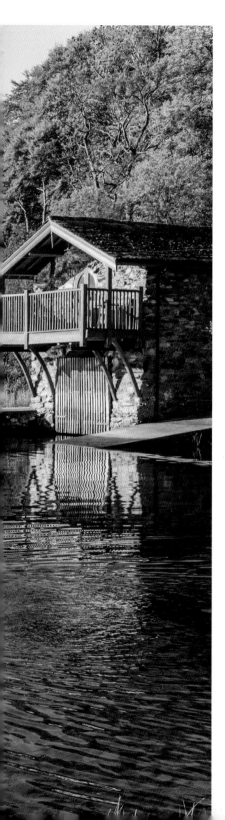

CHAPTER 5

A YEAR IN OUTDOOR SWIMMING

Each season offers outdoor swimmers a different experience, from lazy summer sunset swims to misty morning sunrises in autumn, crisp winter swims followed by shivers and giggles, and spring dips with waterways and shorelines bursting with new life. Strange as it might seem when you start, outdoor swimming really is a year-round activity.

WHY YOU SHOULD SWIM OUTSIDE 365 DAYS OF THE YEAR

When I first started swimming outside regularly in the UK, I thought it was something I might do for three or four months of the year, in a wetsuit. I might have extended that to a little bit of non-wetsuit bodysurfing while on holiday in August in Cornwall. I never imagined it might be something I do 365 days of the year. But some people have always done this.

When you swim in an indoor heated pool, little changes. The main thing I notice is the direction of the sunlight squeezing through the narrow windows. Outdoors, every day of every season offers something different. Outdoor swimming brings you closer to nature than any other sporting activity I know, and it's amazing to experience and observe the changes brought by the seasons from the water.

Obviously, your experience of swimming through the year will vary based on where you live and what access you have to the water. For example, I know of people in the north of England and Scotland who break the ice in order to dip in winter. In some parts of the world, they take chainsaws to frozen lakes and rivers to cut their way into the water below. In other places, winter water temperatures may only fall to the low teens in Celsius (mid-50s in Fahrenheit) and the locals complain that it's too cold. At the coast, the range in water temperatures may be smaller, but you will have days when the water is too wild for swimming. The coldest water I've swum in was around 2°C (35.6°F). I've not yet had the chance to break the ice to swim, but I hope to one day.

In this chapter, we explore some of the things to look out for and enjoy throughout the year. The next chapter, on winter swimming, covers acclimatisation and the practical aspects of dealing with cold water, which is essential reading if you want to be a year-round outdoor swimmer.

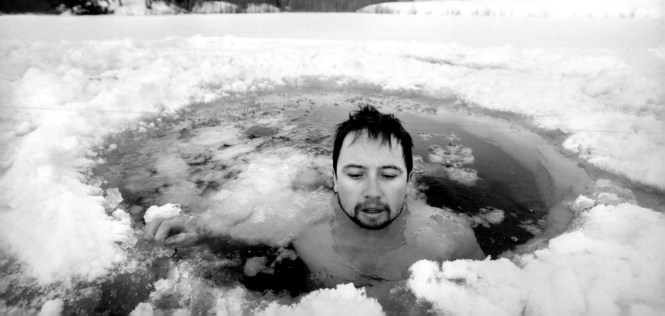

Swimming in Spring

While increasing numbers of commercial venues now offer year-round outdoor swimming, those that don't tend to reopen in April and May. For seasonal swimmers, spring is the time to bring the wetsuit or swimming costume out of storage and closely monitor the weather and water temperatures to decide when to take that first dip of the year. Late spring is always an exciting time for those of us who like to race or take on swimming challenges. The first events of the season typically take place in May and early June in Northern Europe.

Meanwhile, the year-round swimmers, many of them without wetsuits, will be gradually increasing the time they stay in the water as it warms up. Lakes and rivers warm up first, with the sea following a few weeks later. The water temperature in shallow inland waters can vary rapidly. A few days of sunshine might bring a southern UK lake up to 13–14°C (55.4–57.2°F) at the end April, only for it to fall again to single digits after a couple of late frosts in early May. Beware, as this makes a big difference both to your comfort in the water and to your safety.

I love swimming in shallow lakes in spring, especially when they've gained some warmth. The water is often at its clearest and the pond weed hasn't yet had time to grow. The water feels fresh and clean; it isn't too cold but it has a bite to remind you of the winter chill.

The water temperature can also change rapidly in rivers during the spring. Many rivers carry a high silt load that water movement prevents from settling, so the clarity rarely matches what you might find in lakes, especially in spring. I've swum in rivers where you can barely see your hand in front of your face or the person swimming next to you.

Aside from the variable clarity, river swimming in the spring is a joy. Sunrise is still late enough that you can experience it from the water without getting up desperately early. Where I swim, water birds, particularly coots, are busy collecting twigs and building their straggly nests. If you know where to look, you might spot the Canada geese incubating their eggs, which are among the first to hatch. Young swans gather in large (and sometimes intimidating) groups, their grey baby feathers often still showing beneath the white adult ones. Later, you'll see ducklings, cootlings and cygnets. Along the bank, trees blossom. Then, after a windy night, the water will be covered in petals that you can gently push aside as you swim through them.

Down at the coast, the water at the beginning of spring will be close to the coldest it gets. By mid- to late spring, it will be warming up again. Not so many flock to the coast at this time of year, so it's a good time to go if you like the beach to yourself. However, remember that most beaches are not lifeguarded until later in the year.

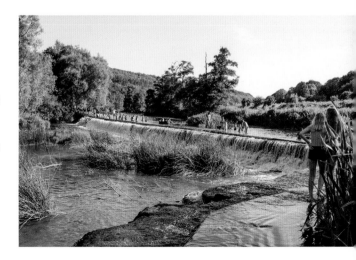

Swimming in Summer

Long evenings, warm water, picnics by the riverside, trips to the seaside: summer has lots to offer swimmers. It's when many people start, drawn to the water to cool off. It's the busiest time for events, the bulk of which take place between June and September. I've often done races on consecutive weekend days and mid-week, too. Most summers I'll do something swimming related every weekend: a race, a family trip to a swim spot, a long swim in a river or the sea with friends.

Inland water temperatures peak in July and August. The Thames frequently reaches the high teens and I once measured it at 24°C (75.2°F). Local lakes see similar temperatures. Further north, it's cooler, but I've swum in Windermere, in the Lake District, at 18°C (64.4°F). Factors such as rainfall, depth and incoming streams and rivers all influence water temperatures, so do be aware that bodies of water in similar locations may have very different temperatures. For example, in Scotland, Loch Ness is connected to Loch Oich by about 8km (5 miles) of canal, yet the former – at least when I swam in both on the same day – is several degrees cooler in summer.

Keep in mind that even 24°C (75.2°F) is cooler than an indoor heated pool, which will typically be kept at 28-31°C (82.4-87.8°F). Stepping into open water always feels cold if you're used to pool temperatures and there is a risk of cold water shock, especially on hot days in earlier summer before the water has warmed up. The sunshine and air temperature may tempt you to strip off and plunge in, but always enter the water carefully and allow your body to adjust.

You should be able to adapt quickly to natural water temperatures in summer. Most people can swim comfortably in UK waters in the summer either with or without a wetsuit. However, be aware you can still become hypothermic, even on a hot day, if you stay in too long. I once took part in a 10km (6.2-mile) swim in Paris. The water was 21°C (69.8°F) and the air about 29°C (84.2°F). I'd travelled light and didn't have a wetsuit with me, but wasn't anticipating any problem with the temperature. However, I started feeling cold over the last few kilometres and struggled to finish, taking nearly an hour longer for the swim than I anticipated. Despite the heat of the day, I ended up spending an hour wrapped in blankets in the medical tent rewarming afterwards.

Summer is a great time to explore wild swimming spots, too, although popular ones may get crowded on hot days. As water temperature changes more slowly than air temperature, it's almost as warm in the water on cloudy days as sunny ones, and often a lot less crowded. If you prefer to avoid the crowds, pick cloudy days or go early in the morning.

Commercial venues are busiest in early summer before people go off on holiday and when triathletes are in full training mode. Luckily, most have plenty of space in the water so they never feel as crowded as swimming pools often do. At the sea, the beaches may be packed and parking can be a nightmare, but there's always space in the water. Go early if you can.

There are a few things to look out for with summer swimming. Waterways are busier on hot days and summer weekends and, depending on where you swim, you may have to share the water with others. As swimmers, we are the most vulnerable people in the water, so always make sure you're visible. Watch out for inexperienced and possibly inebriated boaters who might not expect to find swimmers in the water. I've heard from swimmers who have had close shaves with jetskis and have even encountered them in places where they are not supposed to go. Stay vigilant and look for boat-free swim areas.

Inland, water plants grow quickly, often reaching the water's surface. Some, such as water lilies, are pretty to look at and easy to avoid as long as they don't cover the entire surface. Others seem to reach to just below the surface and you don't see them until you swim into them. They don't pull you down but they can scratch your arms and legs as you untangle yourself. Algae growth reduces visibility in the water. It's mostly harmless (and it's fun to watch the specks swirling in the sunlight under the water), but avoid water with blue-green algae blooms as these are toxic. In the sea, watch out for jellyfish, whose numbers and size typically increase through the summer.

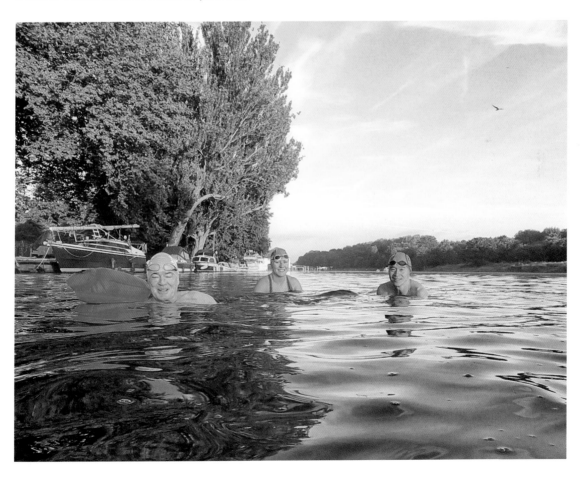

Swimming in Autumn

Autumn brings mixed feelings. As the days shorten and the water cools, you feel the carefree swims of summer slipping away. One of your swims will be your last long outdoor swim of the year. If you like events, they come to an end in the last weeks of September or early October in the UK (some years I've slipped away to southern Europe for a final race of the season in November, which is always a treat). Venues close or switch to shorter winter opening hours around the end of September or early October. Many swimmers stop swimming outdoors in October and do all their swimming in the pool over winter. It's suddenly a lot quieter.

On the other hand, you may be excited by the water cooling down. Given that outdoor swimming's well-being-boosting benefits appear to increase as the water gets colder, continuing your swims may help if you suffer from seasonal affective disorder. Swimming through autumn and gradually getting used to colder water is the best way to prepare for winter.

In my experience, autumn sunrise swims are the most spectacular. As the water cools more slowly than the air, you often have mist rising from the water in the morning. Combine that with the autumn colours and the sun low on the horizon, lighting up a few clouds from underneath, and you have one of life's special moments.

In the sea, in some places, September is the warmest month. The average water temperature in Brighton in September is 17.4ºC (63.3ºF) according to www.seatemperature.org. In August, the next warmest month, it's 17.3ºC (63.1ºF). October is the third-warmest month at 16.3ºC (61.3ºF) and November at 14.5ºC (58.1ºF) is warmer than June, which is 13.8ºC (56.8ºF). An autumn half-term trip to the seaside for some end-of-season swimming might be something to add to your to-do list.

If you're stopping outdoor swimming for the year, give your wetsuit a good wash and make sure it's properly dry before packing it away for winter. Check the rest of your kit, such as tow floats, before putting them away and pack carefully so you don't damage anything.

If, on the other hand, you want to continue swimming outdoors, it's time to start assembling your winter swimming kit, and planning when and where to swim. Find, if you can, some like-minded people who are willing to swim into the colder months with you. There will be times when it's cold, wet and windy, and you won't want to leave your bed. But if you've agreed to meet someone for a swim, you're more likely to get up and go, and you may well have the most amazing time despite the conditions. Or because of them.

The first year I swam through autumn with the intention of swimming into winter, I remember shivering on the bank on a morning in November after a short swim. The water was around 11 or 12ºC (51.8–53.6ºF), and I was feeling pleased with my efforts and saying how this winter swimming thing wasn't as hard as I thought it would be. The person I was swimming with, who had much more experience of these things than me, said: 'I hate to break it to you, but it's not yet winter.'

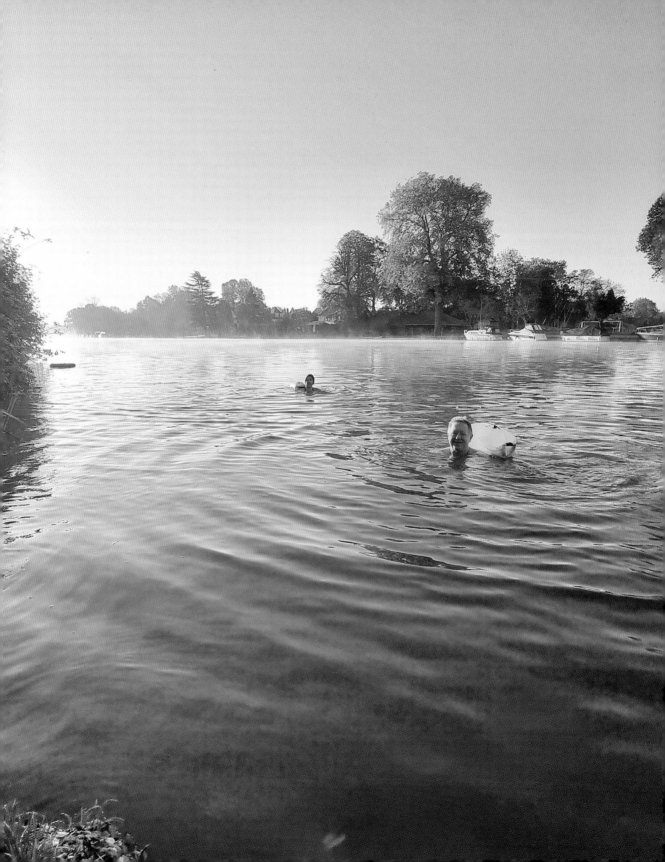

Swimming in Winter

Many swimmers will tell you that winter swimming is when the real magic happens. This is when the water is cold enough to give your body the full cold shock response and the resultant flood of hormones that can be a complete mood changer. Nothing quite anchors in you in the moment like stepping into near-freezing water and then swimming.

While winter swimming gets easier with practice, it takes courage and willpower every time you do it. In this sense, every swim, however short, is a personal victory and confidence booster. There's something satisfying, once you've swum in icy water, about knowing that you could, if you wanted, swim anywhere at any time.

You need a different mindset for winter swimming. For many years I refused to do it on the basis that it was impossible to swim long enough to get any fitness benefit. A swim for me had to be at least 45 minutes and a couple of kilometres to be worth the effort. The option of dressing head to toe in neoprene to try to withstand the cold long enough for a proper training swim was also impractical and unappealing (and still is for me, although some swimmers do it). I know many people still think like this. They're missing the point. Or they get the point, but have other priorities, and that's obviously fine. A five-minute dip doesn't look good on Strava and Garmin doesn't record if you're having fun.

The value in winter swimming is not fitness – at least, not high-end performance fitness – it's in your general health and well-being, and in having fun and mini adventures in the water. It's more social, too. You tend to spend more time changing and chatting than swimming. Sharing a coffee with your fellow swimmers, while you're all layered up in ridiculous amounts of clothes but still shivering, is a definite bonding experience.

And while those who live by training metrics don't see the value of 10 minutes in the water, the cold certainly sends your heart racing. Also, if it does boost your immune system, that could help you be more consistent with other training by reducing time off thanks to colds.

The swimming itself is special, too. As tropical land mammals, swimming in icy water should be totally alien to us. But somehow it isn't, once you've overcome the initial mental and physical barriers. For a brief period, before the cold truly sets in, the water feels amazing. The sun, on the rare days it shines, sits low on the horizon, adding interesting shadows and contrasts to your view. In early winter, the water may still be full of leaf debris, but that clears as winter moves on. As the water temperature drops, you may get excited about how low it will go. What was once impossible becomes possible.

Winter then gives you two special days to swim outdoors: Christmas and New Year. For some people, these might be the only days in winter when they swim outside. If you're tempted to join a festive dip, you'll probably enjoy it more if you've acclimatised first. Remember to save any alcohol until after you've finished swimming and warmed up.

As the winter moves on, the sea continues to get colder, all the way until March. Inland, the coldest water temperatures are usually in January. As the days start getting longer in February, a couple of days of sunshine can make a noticeable difference. It's a relief to leave the finger-numbing sub-5°C (41°F) days behind.

In the next chapter, we explore winter swimming, and how to make the most of it in more detail.

MY STORY

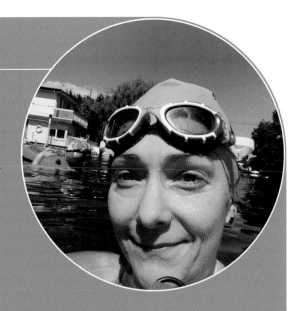

Escapism into obsession

I lose myself when I am in water, in a good way. The feeling of gliding through water is indescribable. I love everything about it, even the cold ... especially the cold.

I was always a swimmer growing up in South Africa and as far as I can remember I always felt like every race ended too soon. However, I quit when I moved into high school, so I never got the opportunity to do the really long races.

As an adult, swimming helps relieve the constant pain I have from a knee injury and a job that keeps me on my feet all day. Water seemed to be the thing I would turn to for support, and I discovered open water and long distance when making one of the biggest decisions of my life.

A few years ago, finding sobriety (not for me, but for someone I loved) gave me a lot of free time at weekends. Waking up when we would have normally been going to sleep, I realised how much I loved feeling good every day of the week. When I found Tooting Bec Lido, I would swim for hours and sometimes more than once a day, just to stay away from my life at home.

Then, in 2014, a friend mentioned the Bournemouth Pier to Pier Swim. It was my first open water race – or at least it felt like a race to me. Up at the crack of dawn and walking down to the beach, I was nervous and excited. This was totally the new high and I loved it. Meanwhile, my partner had hardly slept and could only think about going to the pub. This was the turning point for me.

I finished that event before my friends had walked from Bournemouth to Boscombe. Safe to say, I was totally hooked and a mile wasn't enough. Bring on the English Channel in 2023.

JULIE HACKET

Guide to natural water temperatures

Temperature (ºC)	Description	Comments
>35ºC (>95ºF)	Spa or bath	Too hot for swimming. You'll only experience these temperatures in hot springs or in extreme climates. A bath is typically 40–45ºC (104–113ºF). Dip and soak up the warmth, but don't exert yourself.
30–35ºC (86–95ºF)	Hydrotherapy pool	The sea temperature exceeds 30ºC (86ºF) for a few months of the year in the Persian Gulf, but you won't find these temperatures often in open water. Hydrotherapy pools can be heated to around 32–36ºC (89.6–96.8ºF). Take it easy if you swim and drink plenty of cool water to minimise the risk of heatstroke.
25–30ºC (77–86ºF)	Indoor pool	Indoor pools are typically heated to between 28 and 31ºC (82.4–87.8ºF). Some competition pools are kept at 26ºC (78.8ºF), which feels cool if you're used to regular pools. These temperatures may be reached in extreme weather conditions in shallow UK lakes. Don't wear a wetsuit.
20–25ºC (68–77ºF)	Warm	Occasionally reached in shallower lakes during hot spells in temperate climates. If you're a wetsuit wearer, consider removing it in these temperatures, especially at the upper end of the range, to avoid heatstroke. Lengthy non-wetsuit swims in comfort are possible at these temperatures.
15–20ºC (59–68ºF)	Moderate	Sea temperatures around the UK typically top out in the high teens in August and September. Once acclimatised, many people can swim comfortably in these temperatures. For elite marathon swimming events, wetsuits are optional below 20ºC (68ºF) and compulsory below 18ºC (64.4ºF). Elite marathon swimming races should not go ahead below 16ºC (60.8ºF), although other events can.
10–15ºC (50–59ºF)	Cold	Unacclimatised people will get a significant cold water shock response in this range, especially towards the lower end. Wetsuits are compulsory in triathlon below 14ºC (57.2ºF) and swimming in UK triathlon events is not permitted below 11ºC (51.8ºF). Short non-wetsuit swims and longer wetsuit swims are manageable for most people at these temperatures.
5–10ºC (41º–50ºF)	Extreme cold	Below 10ºC (50ºF) is winter swimming territory. Sea temperatures around the UK are often in this range in the winter. Water below about 8ºC (46.4ºF) triggers pain sensors, so you feel pain from the water as well as cold, with your feet, hands and face being the most sensitive. Keep your swims short.
0–5ºC (32–41ºF)	Icy	Since the invention of the 'Ice Mile', a mile swum in water of less than 5ºC (41ºF), that temperature has become something of a benchmark for winter swimmers. Inland lakes and rivers can plunge this low in winter. Icy water can cause significant pain in your hands, feet and face. Keep your swims under 10 minutes.
<0ºC (<32ºF)		As fresh water freezes at 0ºC (32ºF), you won't find sub-zero water inland, but you may come across it in the sea as salt water can stay liquid until about -1.8ºC (28.8ºF). However, body tissue starts freezing at -0.6ºC (30.9ºF). Swimming in these temperatures is usually only done for records and extreme swim challenges, and must be fully supervised by experts and swim safety professionals.

The ranges in the table opposite are basic guidelines only. There are significant differences between the top and bottom temperatures in these ranges, and swimmers feel and are affected by every degree of change in water temperature. These can be seen, for example, by looking at the wetsuit rules set by the Fédération Internationale De Natation (FINA) for elite open water competition. FINA, which is the international federation for swimming, based its rules primarily on research carried out at the Extreme Environments Laboratory (EEL) at the University of Portsmouth. The EEL monitored changes in swimmers' core body temperature while they swam in a flume at various temperatures. Based on those findings, FINA concluded that wetsuits must be worn below 18ºC (64.4ºF) and are not needed above 20ºC (68ºF) in events sanctioned by them.

I once took part in a study on the effects of cool water and swam for two hours in the flume at 16ºC (60.8ºF). Two weeks later, I returned and did the same thing at 18ºC (64.4ºF). On the first swim, I was cold and miserable throughout and by the end my core temperature had dropped to 36.3ºC (97.3ºF). It then continued dropping for a further 30 minutes, reaching 35.6ºC (96ºF) before recovering. On the second swim, I felt comfortable throughout. My temperature only dropped to 37ºC (98.6ºF) by the end of the swim and bottomed out at 36.3ºC (97.3ºF) during the 30-minute post-swim recovery. A mere 2ºC (3.6ºF) difference in water temperature brought me much closer to hypothermia, which is usually defined as a core body temperature of less than 35ºC (95ºF).

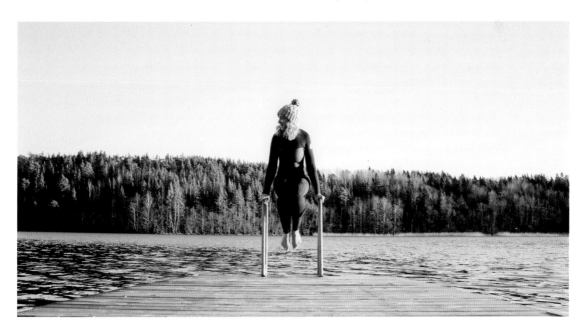

OUTDOOR SWIMMING AND DISABILITY

Swimming outside in natural waters challenges everyone. For swimmers with disabilities, some of those challenges are magnified. Yet swimmers with disabilities describe the same positive feelings and get the same benefits from outdoor swimming as anyone else. Sometimes they sound even more positive.

Sophie Etheridge has been a wheelchair user since she was involved in a cycling accident when she was 19. Before the accident, she was a physically active teenager and a competitive swimmer. It took her five years from the accident before she swam in open water again. 'There were so many barriers to overcome and I had no one to help me,' she says.

Questions she needed answering before she could swim included practical considerations such as the availability of disabled car parking spaces, the distance from the car park to the water and what type of terrain she'd have to cross. And that's before she even got to the water.

If she's visiting a commercial venue or taking part in an event, she wonders if there will be disabled changing rooms and where she can leave her wheelchair. How will she get into the water? Is there a beach or a ramp she can shuffle down or is it steps?

As Sophie explored getting back into swimming, she quickly realised the barriers were not just practical and physical, they were also mental. She explained how, when she first got back into the water, she wanted to swim like she could before the accident and it took time to adjust to a new way of swimming. She also felt undignified shuffling into and out of the water on her bottom and was embarrassed by other mishaps and clumsiness resulting from her injuries. It took time to gain confidence and to be able to laugh it off when she has difficulties. She now describes herself as an 'adaptive swimmer' to focus on how she's been able to adapt to achieve the things she wants to.

As well as swimming at commercial venues that have at least some facilities she can use and relatively easy access to the water, Sophie likes to wild swim, which poses additional challenges. One of which is the anxiety that her wheelchair might be stolen while she's in the water. 'I know someone whose prosthetic leg was stolen while they were swimming,' she says. 'I've no idea why – it would be no use to anyone else.'

Once in the water, Sophie describes having a great sense of freedom, both physically and mentally. 'In the water, I'm no longer stuck in my chair. I don't have to worry about uneven paths or sinking in the mud.'

Sophie can walk short distances with the aid of crutches, but it causes her considerable pain. In the water, she can move freely. 'It's a lot easier and a lot less painful than walking,' she says.

On the mental side, she says we live in a very judgemental world for disabled people. In the water, she's at the same level as everyone else. If she meets someone for the first time in a lake, they won't realise she's disabled. 'There's no judgement or questions in people's eyes. It's very rare that you get this. It's not that I'm pretending not to be disabled, it's just a relief sometimes. People can't see the difference between me and anyone else.'

Like almost every outdoor swimmer I speak to, Sophie says the activity has big benefits for her mental health, something she's struggled with at times. 'It gives me space to think and be at peace. Sunset in the lake, in the park, there's nothing else like it. It focuses you on the present moment. On longer swims, I can relax, turn on autopilot and go through things in my head, something I can never do on land.'

After battling on her own to break down barriers to outdoor swimming, Sophie realised she could help others and set up a Facebook group, Adaptive/Disabled Open Water Swimmers (ADOWS) – for swimmers with disabilities to share tips and advice. Within 24 hours she'd received more than 150 requests to join and the group quickly expanded to more than 300 people. Sophie has also trained to become an outdoor swimming coach. You can read more about her journey on her website. This also hosts another project she's working on: a map of accessible swimming spots.

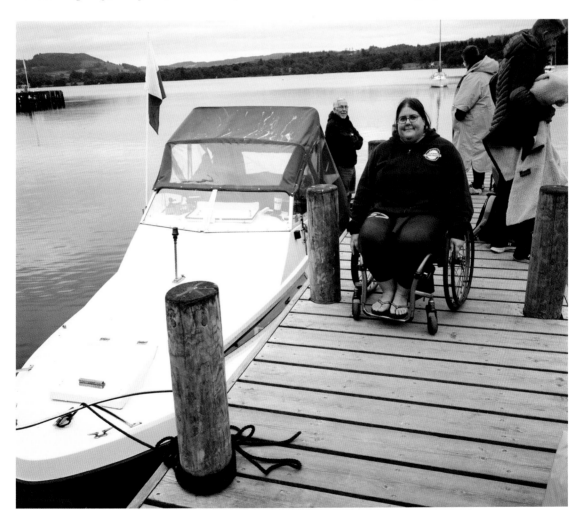

Sophie's top tips on swimming with a disability

1. Every swimmer and every disability is different. You may need to use trial and error to find what works for you.

2. Feel free to experiment. Sophie used to put a band around her ankles to help keep her legs from drifting apart. Some swimmers use floatation belts for additional buoyancy.

3. Test any new kit or ideas in a pool before bringing them to the open water.

4. Try not to worry about how you swim or get into or out of the water. Just do it however you can.

5. If you have a MedicAlert, keep it with you while you swim.

6. When starting out, swim at a venue that has full safety cover.

7. Always swim with someone else.

8. If you're going to a new venue or taking part in an event, contact the organiser in advance to discuss your requirements.

9. Listen to your body. Swimmers with disabilities are often very in tune with how they feel. However, with some conditions it may be difficult to tell if you are getting too cold, for example. Take time to understand how your body reacts when outdoor swimming, especially in cold water. Keep your swims short to start with.

10. Join the Adaptive/Disabled Open Water Swimmers group on Facebook.

MY STORY

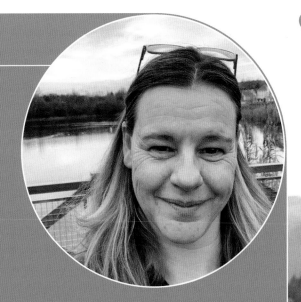

Swimming without barriers

I have been a passionate swimmer since a friend took me to the pool when I was 10. I soon started training twice a day and made it to the South African National Championships, where I won a relay medal and finished in the top 15 over 50m (55 yards) freestyle. Being profoundly deaf since birth, I went to the Deaflympics in 1993 and won one gold and three silver medals.

Having experienced the rewards of a life in sport, but also having to overcome significant obstacles due to my deafness, I wanted to do something to make sport more accessible to deaf people. As part of that, and now living in the UK, I decided to become an open water swimming coach and created my own business (Swimming Without Barriers) that offers coaching services, outdoor swimming workshops and swimming holidays.

CAROLINE HURLEY

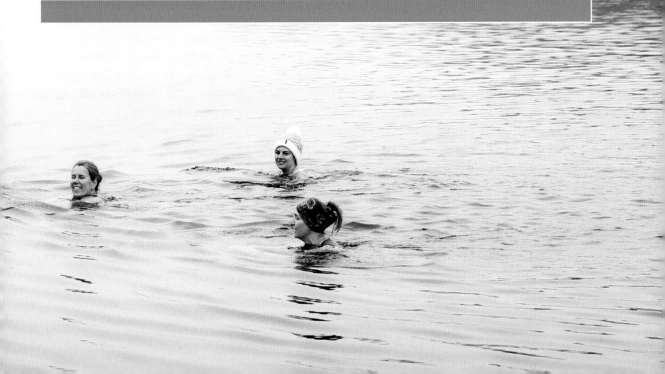

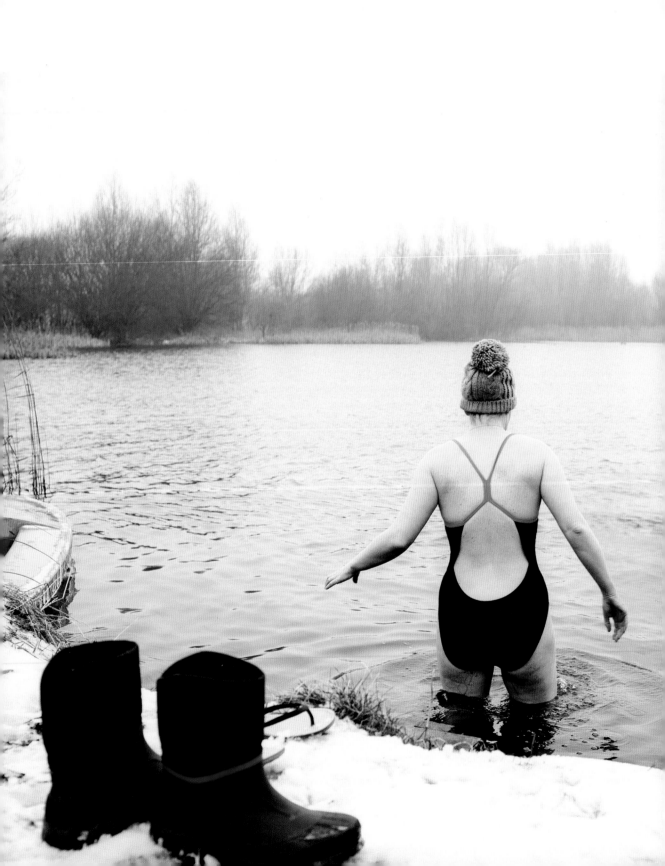

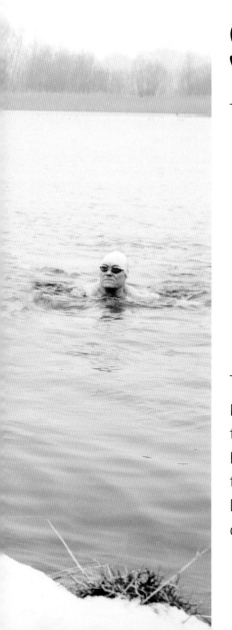

CHAPTER 6

WINTER AND COLD WATER SWIMMING

Discover more about why you should embrace the cold and consider swimming outside in winter. Find out how and where to get started, and how to warm up again afterwards. We also take a look at eccentric but sociable winter swimming competitions and the daunting Ice Mile.

HOW TO EMBRACE THE COLD

Yes, cold water is scary. It can cause short-term pain and it's dangerous if you stay in too long. But it's also magical. To enjoy its benefits, you need to see past your fears and natural aversion and embrace the cold.

There is no formal definition for winter swimming. It's linked neither to the astronomical definition of winter, which in the northern hemisphere is roughly 21 December to 20 March, nor to the meteorological definition of winter, 1 December to the last day in February. How about we agree that winter swimming is swimming outside in natural water temperatures between the dates the clocks change to mark the end and beginning of daylight saving hours (if applicable)?

There is no agreed definition of cold water swimming. Water at 15ºC (59ºF) is cold enough to induce cold water shock and certainly feels cold, but some extreme swimmers don't think it's cold unless it's less than 5ºC (41ºF). I'd suggest below 15ºC (59ºF) is a good starting point for beginners. I also think 10ºC (50ºF) is a nice memorable benchmark. But feel free to have your own definition of cold and adjust it depending on your mood and experience.

As a recent convert to winter swimming, please forgive me if I write about it with the zeal of an evangelist. If I were writing this a few years ago, I would have advised you to avoid it, and my experience of it would have been mostly vicarious. But now, having swum outside all winter due to Covid-19-related pool closures, I can honestly recommend giving it a go. I can see it's not for everyone, but don't dismiss it without trying it.

Prior to my winter of swimming, my few feeble attempts amounted to the following:

• Wading into Windermere up to my thighs, in February, and refusing to go any further because of the pain.
• Being volunteered to take part in a fancy-dress cold water relay at Tooting Bec Lido with the *Outdoor Swimmer* team. I managed my single 30m (33-yard) width, dressed as Batman, because there was no way to chicken out, and it was awful. I was in the water for less than 45 seconds.
• Convincing two of my children, then aged 10 and 12, to come to Tooting Bec Lido with me in winter. We all swam a width. I'm not sure if they've ever forgiven me.
• Entering a cold water swimming event in Windermere for journalistic research and trying to swim 60m (66 yards) front crawl. I managed it, but was shocked at how hard it was to breathe and I couldn't put my face in the water.

The problem with all of these attempts was that I hadn't acclimatised. I couldn't get my head around the idea that just a few dips significantly reduces the cold water shock response. Nor could I understand how people could possibly be comfortable in near-freezing water. I assumed that some people were different and could just cope better with cold. I now know it's relatively easy to adapt. But before we look at how to do that, what about the question of wetsuits?

Should you wear a wetsuit for winter swimming?

Yes	No
While a wetsuit doesn't prevent cold water shock, it can reduce the response as your skin has some protection from the cold water. The wetsuit then keeps you warmer, reducing the risk of swim failure and hypothermia, and allowing you to swim for longer. A wetsuit also increases your buoyancy, making it almost impossible to sink.	For the true cold water experience, it's best to feel the water directly against the skin. Wearing a wetsuit also seems to make your exposed parts (hands, feet and face) suffer more from the cold than when you go without. Once you finish swimming, you can dress immediately and warm up quicker if you're not wearing a wetsuit, and you don't have the hassle of washing and drying it either.

Recommendation: Try both and see which you like best.

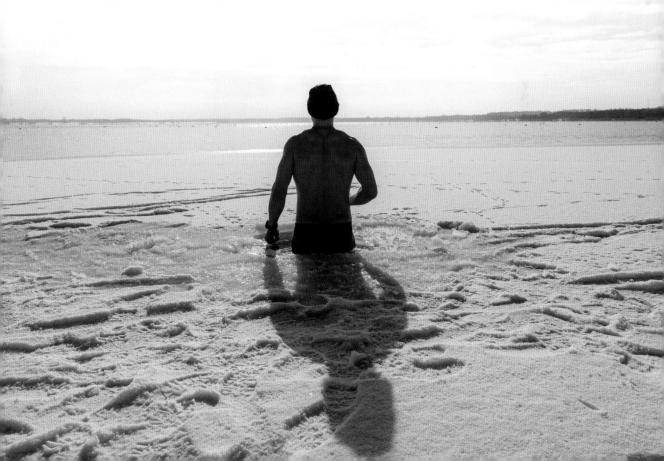

RECREATIONAL WINTER SWIMMING

Winter swimming is a great leveller and is therefore often very social. The shared experience of getting into the water is more important than your speed through the water. A lot of people swim head-up breaststroke, stick together and chat, rather than putting their faces in the water and trying to swim fast.

When to start

The easiest way to adapt to winter swimming is to start in the summer and keep going as the water cools down. This way, you gain experience of outdoor swimming in the warmer and safer conditions of summer and give yourself plenty of time to adapt. This is the way I did it. But you don't have to. Jonathan Cowie, the editor at *Outdoor Swimmer* magazine, started on Christmas Day.

Whenever you take the plunge, keep the following in mind

- Despite all the benefits of cold water, it can be dangerous. Make sure you familiarise yourself with the risks.
- The cold water shock response and phase of maximum discomfort lasts for about one to two minutes. It gets more comfortable and enjoyable after that.
- The cold shock response diminishes significantly after a handful of immersions. Once you've done it a few times, getting in becomes easier.
- The cold water shock response doesn't appear to get any stronger as temperatures drop below 10ºC (50ºF). However, your adaptation is only to the temperatures you have swum in. If you've only adapted to 10ºC (50ºF), you will get cold water shock at 5°C (41ºF).

- Provided that you start warm, and get dressed and warm immediately afterwards, you will not get hypothermia at any temperature with swims that last less than 10 minutes. Keep your swims short.
- You get most of the benefits of cold water swimming from the first few minutes of immersion. Longer swims increase the risk, not the benefits, which is another reason to keep your swims short.
- Always swim with other people or where there are lifeguards who can provide assistance if necessary.

MY STORY

Triathlete turned winter swimmer

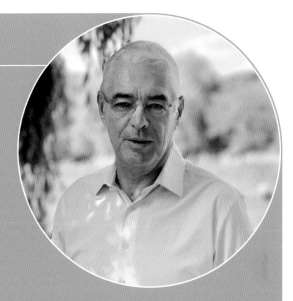

There is heavy frost on the ground, the air temperature is -4ºC (24.8ºF) and I'm swooshing down the swollen, murky Thames, whooping and swearing in equal measure. My hands and feet are in serious pain and I know I can't get out of the water until the exit point 500m (550 yards) downriver. Luckily, given the speed of the current, that should only take a few minutes to reach, but how did I end up here, in 3ºC (37.4ºF) water on New Year's Day 2021?

Before Covid-19, I could not have imagined myself ever swimming in the Thames, never mind going 'skins' all through the winter in ever-decreasing temperatures and looking forward to every outing with a nervous anticipation. I wasn't a stranger to open water swimming, but that was almost exclusively in the warm seas of South East Asia. I caught the triathlon bug 13 years ago, learned to swim and had a great 10 years racing around the Middle East and Asia in my 50s until an ankle injury killed off the running part and almost the cycling, too.

After 33 years living and working around the world, I landed in Twickenham in 2017. During the 2020 summer of Covid-19, I joined up with a group of fast-swimming wetsuited swimmers for regular swims up and down the Thames. Little did I know that by autumn we would dump the wetsuits and keep swimming, even if at times we could only swim in socially distanced pairs.

For me, it was about doing something to keep active during the lockdowns. I have always liked some risk in my life and this cold water skins stuff with the unpredictable flow rate and the ice-block hands and feet really did suit me.

If the pools had been open, would I have done it? Actually, I think so. Either way, the winter of 2020 was very special in one way during the lockdowns and I won't forget it.

ANDREW O'REGAN

Where to Swim

You can winter swim in almost all the same places that you swim in the summer. Unheated lidos, while not true 'open water', deserve special mention as the safest places for a cold water swimming experience. Increasing numbers now stay open throughout the winter or have extended their opening season further into autumn to cater to the growing demand for winter swimming. Even so, opening hours are often restricted, so check before you swim. In some cases, the pools may be closed for general swimming, but still allow local clubs or swimming groups to meet. These are worth looking out for and joining.

As well as lidos, increasing numbers of commercial swimming venues now stay open through winter, again often on restricted opening times or only for clubs or groups.

For free winter swimming options, you'll need to head to the coast or find a river or lake where swimming is allowed, as in summer. The same groups you find in those places often meet up for winter swimming, too, so it's well worth searching online and social media and trying to connect with one.

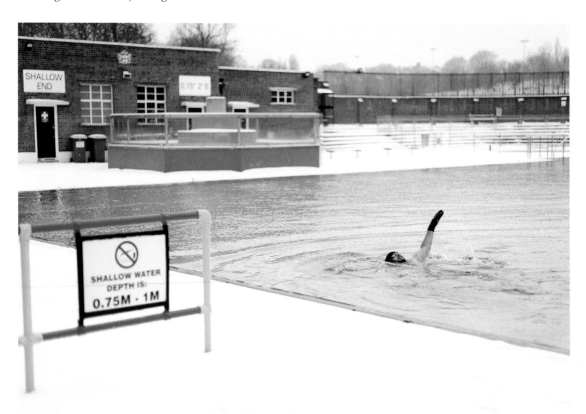

How to Start

I know I keep repeating this, but the risks of swimming in winter are much higher than in summer, so please read the safety chapter again and start cautiously. A winter dip needs more planning than a summer swim. There is less scope for spontaneity. You have to think through and organise how you will warm up afterwards, before you get in the water.

Cold water swimming kit checklist

- Clothes you can pull on quickly (avoid buttons and fiddly zips).
- Changing mat (an old groundsheet will do).
- Warm hat, gloves and scarf.
- Thick socks.
- Slip-on shoes or fleece-lined boots.
- Winter coat and/or changing robe.
- Warm drink in a flask.
- Hot water bottle.
- Two towels (one to stand on).
- Waterproof bag.

Make sure you know exactly where and how you will get in and out of the water before you change. Check for any hazards, such as slippery rocks, currents or sudden changes in depth, so you can prepare for them.

Try to stay warm before you swim. Only undress when it's time to swim. I usually go to a winter swim already wearing my costume beneath my clothes to minimise undressing time. Some swimmers put on their swimming cap and goggles (if they're using them) before undressing, again to reduce the amount of time between when you have removed your clothes and when you enter the water.

As you change, stack your clothes in the order you will put them on afterwards. Make sure they are the right way around. I like to wrap mine around a hot water bottle to pre-warm them. This also prevents them blowing away if it's windy. I prefer to have at least two more layers to the number I'd be comfortable in pre swim.

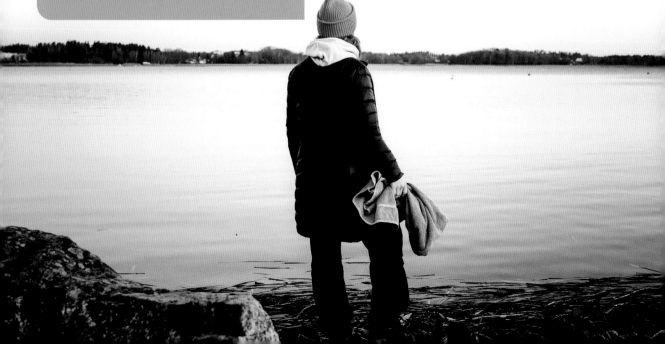

Top tip for men
Only use a single knot to tie your trunks and leave the cord looser than you would for a regular swim. This helps avoid the embarrassment of having to ask someone else to unknot your trunks if your fingers have got too numb to do it yourself.

Top tip for women
Apparently, when your skin is cold and damp, and your fingers are numb, the easiest thing to put on is another swimming costume, so you can avoid the hassle of trying to clip a bra.

Before you enter the water, remind yourself that the first couple of minutes are the hardest because of cold water shock. Some people like to splash water on their face and neck to reduce the cold water shock response. I'd rather just get in, but do what feels right for you. Get in purposefully and lower yourself until your shoulders are covered. Breathe out. Take whatever time you need at this stage. Some experienced swimmers can safely and comfortably start swimming immediately, but it's essential to ensure your breathing is under control and that you're not feeling any sense of panic before you continue. You will feel cold. You may feel pain (hands and feet are particularly susceptible). Your heart and breathing rates will have jumped. Tell yourself this is normal and will pass.

When you're ready, lift the weight off your feet and swim. Many people, including me, swim head-up breaststroke in cold water as it minimises that ice-cream headache feeling. Other people seem happy to put their face down and swim front crawl.

Don't venture far. It will start to feel better after one to two minutes, but that might be too long for your first swim. Leave yourself the option of changing your mind.

Once you're through the initial phase and into the 'it-feels-amazing' stage, take care not to overstay your welcome in the water. Set a limit before you start and stick to it. In water of 10ºC (50ºF) or less, I suggest a maximum of 10 minutes, based on advice from researchers at the Extreme Environments Laboratory at the University of Portsmouth. There's no need to stay in longer to receive the benefits of cold water immersion, so why take the risk?

Once you leave the water, your body will continue cooling. If it's windy, you will cool faster. You, on the other hand, will feel indestructible. Cold water does that to you. But don't be fooled. Take advantage of those first couple of minutes to remove your wet costume and pull on as many layers as possible. Start with a hat and the top half of your body. The more you can do before you start shivering or your fingers go numb, the better.

Keep in mind that in winter, the proportion of time devoted to swimming and socialising is inverted. Swimmers usually spend a great deal more time warming up and chatting after a swim than they do in the water. Come prepared with warm clothes, a hot drink and a shareable snack.

The Recovery

When you're in cold water, heat is conducted away from your body into the water, starting with the skin and tissue close to the skin. Once you leave the water, this 'cold front' continues moving through your body and your core temperature keeps falling for about 20–30 minutes. This is why swimmers often start to shiver and feel cold a few minutes after they have left the water. As mentioned previously, swimmers refer to this phenomenon as 'after drop' while scientists prefer the term 'continued cooling'. It's normal and mostly nothing to worry about. The post-swim shivers are part of the fun of winter swimming.

However, your core temperature can drop significantly after leaving the water. In the study I took part in, my temperature dropped by a full 1°C (1.8°F) in the 30 minutes after I finished swimming. It could easily drop more if you don't dress immediately and shelter from the wind. This means you can become hypothermic after your swim, even if you're fine when you leave the water. This is important to remember if you drove or cycled to your swim spot: ensure you allow enough time to rewarm before attempting driving or cycling again. This could be up to an hour if you've become excessively cold and it's another good reason to keep your swims short.

The physics says a hot drink will make a negligible difference to helping you rewarm. The reality is that sipping a warm drink and holding a hot mug in your hands makes you feel better. Be careful not to have it too hot. If you're shivering, you might have trouble connecting mug to mouth, with scalding consequences. Shivering also burns lots of calories so try to eat something too.

Be wary of hot showers until you have warmed up. It's better to dress immediately after swimming, warm up and then shower. You could waste a lot of hot water trying to warm up under a shower and may slow your rewarming by dilating your superficial blood vessels. Moreover, this sudden dilation of blood vessels may cause you to faint due to a drop in blood pressure. A hot water bottle is nice to hug or hold between your legs, but dress first and don't put the hot water bottle directly against your skin.

As long as you have avoided the potential pitfalls of winter swimming, you should now feel good for the rest of the day.

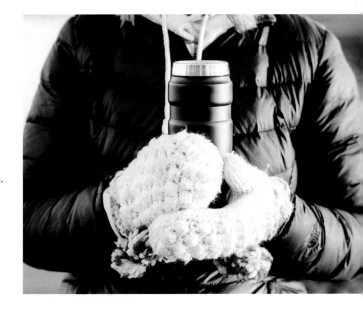

Winter Swimming Competitions

South London Swimming Club (SLSC) has organised a Cold Water Swimming Championships event at Tooting Bec Lido biannually since 2006. The idea for the event came after a group of club members had travelled to northern Finland in 2005 to take part in an ice swimming event. Subsequently, SLSC were asked if they would like to host the World Winter Swimming Championships, which they duly did in 2008. You can find the full story on SLSC's website.

Now, 'championships' sound like serious undertakings. From the organisers' perspective, these events require massive amounts of preparation and planning, and they run with military-like precision. Safety is taken extremely seriously. But for participants, it's mostly fun and often an opportunity to meet like-minded swimmers from around the world. The events are open to anyone. There are no qualifying times or standards for the shorter swims, although longer swims sometimes require entrants to confirm their capabilities. There are often prizes for fancy dress and elaborate hats, which are more keenly contested than any medals for winning races.

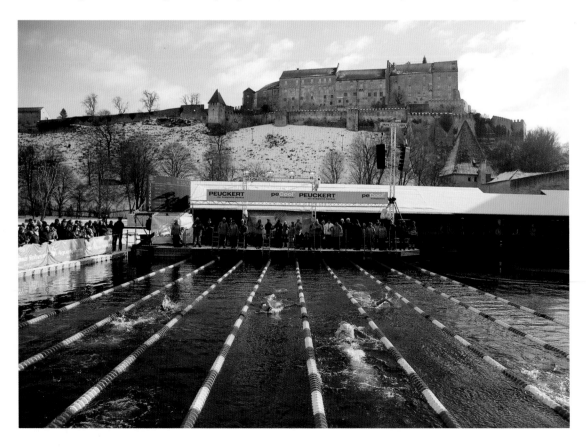

Like school swimming galas, cold water championships events feature a range of races of different distances and strokes, from 25m (27.5 yards) breaststroke to 1000m (1100 yards) freestyle. Prizes are usually awarded in five-year age bands. There are also relays, which may involve fancy dress. Most events provide hot tubs for swimmers to warm up in after their swims.

The strongest traditions for winter swimming are in Scandinavia and Russia but look out also for events in Scotland, Slovenia (in the fairy-tale Lake Bled), Germany and China. The International Winter Swimming Association maintains a list of events plus full details of the rules on its website.

In 2015, I took part in the Big Chill Swim, a winter swimming event in Windermere. Chillswim, the organiser, create a 25m (27.5-yard) 'pool' in the marina opposite the Low Wood Bay hotel. I picked the race that would require the shortest time in the water – the 50m (55 yard) freestyle or two lengths of the pool. I was given a card with the exact time of my swim and precise instructions on where I had to be when. I arrived at the pre-swim muster area fully dressed, with my costume under my clothes. Everything had to be ready for a slick change. Two minutes before the swim, marshals led us out on to the decking and instructed us to stand behind our lanes. We were then told to remove our clothing and enter the water.

Diving is not allowed in winter swimming events and you must get your shoulders under the water before the start signal. It's bad etiquette to keep your fellow swimmers waiting in the water and getting cold, so you need to shed your clothes quickly and lower yourself down the steps into the water at the same time as everyone else. Once everyone had their shoulders below the water, the starter sounded and I swam. I remember keeping my head up and feeling crushed by the cold. At the turn, it was the thought that swimming was the quickest way back to my clothes that kept me going. Tumble turns aren't allowed in winter championship races, but I wouldn't have been able to do one anyway. As soon as I finished, I climbed out of the water, grabbed my clothes and sprinted for the hot tub. I didn't even stop to look where I'd finished.

I only signed up for one race, but many people enter several. While swimming is the reason for being there, the international festival atmosphere and post-swim celebrations are a big draw. People often travel long distances for these IWSA events. True cold water swimming fans happily travel to Siberia in the middle of winter where the air temperature might be -20ºC (-4ºF) and the ice (1m/93.3ft) thick. There's a saying among winter swimmers that the colder the water, the warmer the welcome.

The Ice Mile

Inevitably, as with many activities, some people want to explore their physical and mental limits. Lewis Pugh famously swam 1km (0.62 miles) in -1.7°C (28.9°F) water at the North Pole in 2007. Fresh water freezes at 0°C (32°F), but sea water can get colder before it ices over. Still, the North Pole should be frozen and Pugh did the swim to draw attention to the fact that it wasn't. If you haven't seen it already, it's worth searching out his TED talk about the swim.

While Pugh's polar swim was a unique challenge, the concept of swimming long(ish) distances in icy water has caught on. The International Ice Swimming Association (IISA) was created by South African extreme swimmer Ram Barkai in 2009 to formalise swimming in icy water – which it describes as water of less than 5°C (41°F) – and introduced the Ice Mile. The Ice Mile is defined as swimming a mile (1.6km) in water of 5°C (41°F) or less, in a standard swimming costume, goggles and cap. No wetsuits allowed.

Make no mistake, an Ice Mile is a serious undertaking and an extreme sports event that puts a great deal of strain on your body and carries a high risk of hypothermia. To put it in context, a typical Ice Mile takes between 24 and 50 minutes, although some swimmers have taken more than an hour. In water at this temperature, the United States Search and Rescue Task Force says the typical time to exhaustion or loss of consciousness is between 15 and 30 minutes. The expected survival time (assuming your airways can be kept free and you don't drown) is 30–90 minutes. Nearly everyone who completes an Ice Mile has to stay in the water for longer than the expected time to unconsciousness.

Training, acclimatisation, and body shape and size can all extend the amount of time you can swim in cold water, but you cannot stop the progression to hypothermia at these temperatures. In one Ice Mile that I watched, all swimmers started strongly, but began to slow down as the cold set in. One swimmer showed a classic case of swim failure with his stroke rate slowing and legs sinking until he stopped moving, and needed to be rescued. He subsequently spent a couple of hours recovering from hypothermia in the medical tent. An Ice Mile should only be attempted after lengthy training and acclimatising and when a full safety team is in place in accordance with IISA guidelines.

The IISA (which is a separate organisation to the IWSA) organises and sanctions its own series of ice swimming events focusing on the longer distances of 250m (275 yards), 500m (550 yards) and 1000m (1100 yards). Details are on its website.

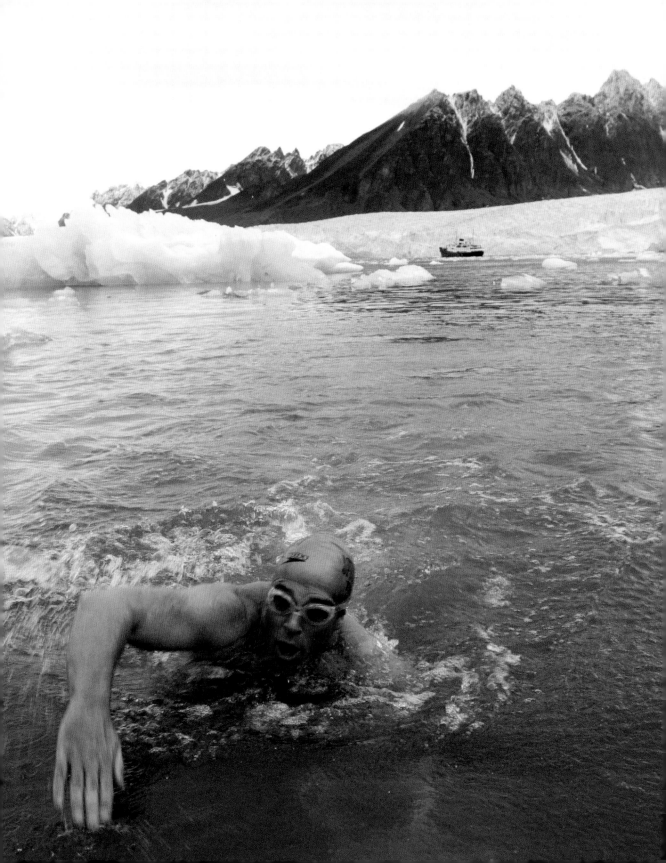

WHAT ABOUT COLD SHOWERS AND ICE BATHS?

You may have seen pictures of people sitting in ice-filled water in paddling pools or wheelie bins or you may have heard people talking about cold showers. Why would anyone do this? Should you? Do I?

One reason people take cold showers and cold baths is to help with acclimatisation. I am not aware of any study that has directly measured if cold showers or ice baths help in the acclimatisation process for swimmers, but it's plausible and I'm sure there must be a psychological benefit. Part of the challenge with entering cold water is mental, and if you've practised in the safety and privacy of your bathroom, it should make it easier outdoors. However, one study looked at differences between static immersion in cold water and swimming, with both acclimatised and non-acclimatised swimmers. While static, the acclimatised swimmers lost heat faster due to a decreased metabolic rate. When they were swimming, they were able to maintain deep body temperature.

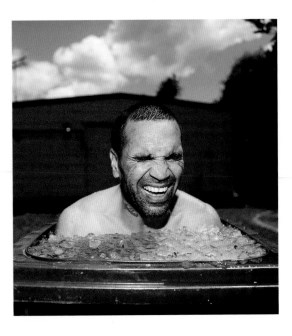

Our bodies thus respond differently to cold water immersion depending on whether we are static or swimming, which suggests that cold baths may not help you to adapt to swimming in cold water, though they should help in controlling your cold water shock response.

A second reason is that cold showers and baths may be good for you in their own right. Cold water immersion doesn't need to be in open water to generate that rush of hormones and spike in your heart rate. An ice bath will do just fine.

Third, some swimmers use language that equates their desire for cold water to that of an addiction. They say they need their cold water fix and if they can't get into the sea, a lake or a river, then a wheelie bin full of icy water will have to do.

Personally, I like the idea of being able to move when I'm in cold water. Blasting myself with cold water from a shower or stepping into a cold bath seems much less appealing than a brief, brisk swim in a river.

If you do try cold showers and especially cold baths, remember you can still get cold water shock or hypothermic in your bathroom, so do take care.

MY STORY

Ice lover

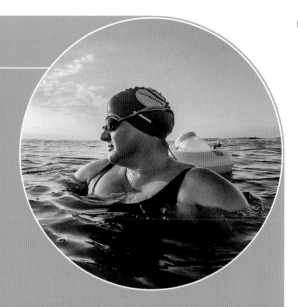

I was always a water baby and often swam in rivers as a child. I was introduced to competitive open water swimming, with a wetsuit, through triathlon. However, it wasn't until I reached 43 that I discovered my true passion: winter swimming. I ditched the wetsuit and never looked back.

Starting in 2015, along with a few friends, I signed up for the Big Chill Swim, a winter swimming event in Windermere. We had no idea what we were getting into, but it sounded bonkers enough to give it a try. As I continued swimming through the autumn leading up to the event, something unexpected happened. I got addicted to the cold water and was going four or five times a week. I just loved it. It became my reset button and the only time I can switch off my hyperactive mind.

Those swims started me on a journey I never even dreamed of. I went on to swim the English Channel, complete eight official Ice Miles and set a world record for the most southerly Ice Mile in Antarctica. Nevertheless, I'm still happiest floating around my local swim spot, Keeper's Pond (or Pen-ffordd-goch Pond) above Blaenavon, with my friends and having a chat, especially when the water temperature drops below 8ºC (46.4ºF). When I swim in warmer water, my mind wanders to all the things I need to do, but when it's cold, I can't think of anything else. It's a real in-the-moment experience. It re-energises me.

CATH PENDLETON

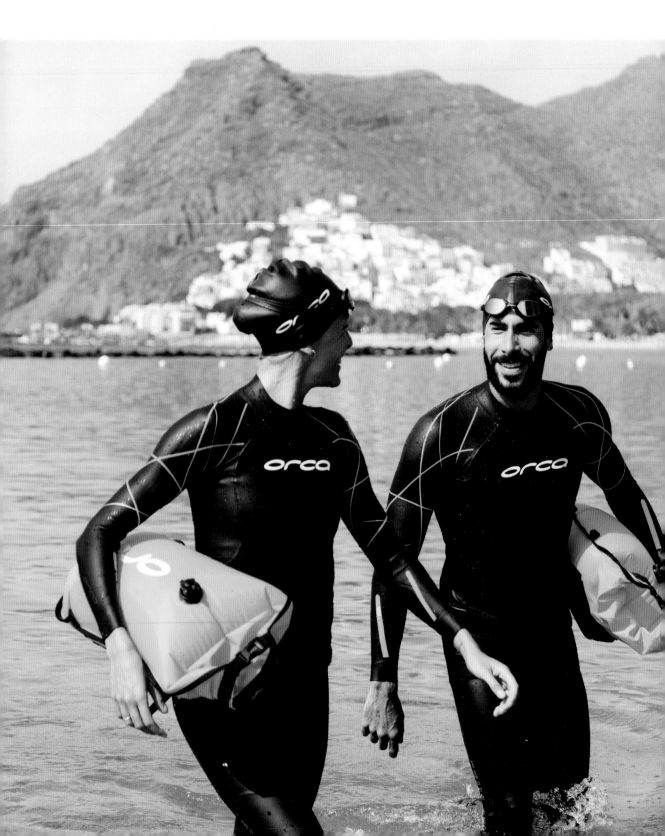

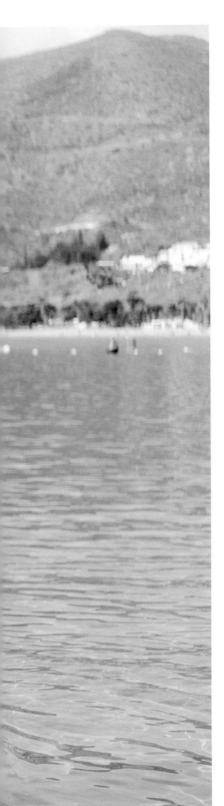

CHAPTER 7

OUTDOOR SWIMMING KIT

What do you need, what's nice to have, what can you do without – and, importantly, how do you use the kit you've got? In this chapter, we dive deep into the fascinating world of stuff for outdoor swimmers. There's more to it than you might think.

KIT ESSENTIALS

You could start outdoor swimming with no kit whatsoever, but having a few well-chosen items will make you more comfortable and improve your safety.

Kit checklist		
	In the water	*Before and after*
Essential	Nothing	Clothes
Recommended	Costume Goggles Swimming hat Tow float or bag	Towel Extra layers Flip-flops or similar Changing robe
Optional	Wetsuit Neoprene accessories Sports watch Waterproof phone pouch Waterproof camera Whistle (for attracting attention)	Changing mat Waterproof kit bag Thermos flask containing a warm drink Snacks Hat, gloves, scarf (winter) Sunscreen (summer)

What Do I Need?

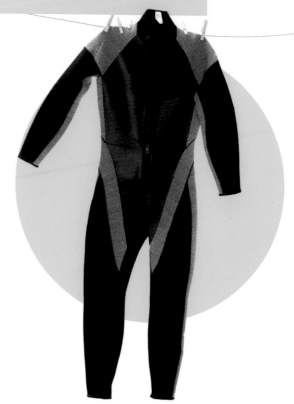

I love the spontaneity of outdoor swimming. If you discover a beautiful place to swim, you can swim, even if you have no kit with you. If it's not private or secluded enough to swim naked, you can take a dip in your underwear. However, having the right kit can make your swims safer and more comfortable. And, let's face it, going home with dripping underwear after a spontaneous dip can be a nuisance.

When buying new kit, as well as cost, check the environmental credentials. Where does it come from? Is the packaging excessive? Is the material recycled or recyclable? If not, will it at least last a long time? Follow the care instructions for any kit you own to maximise its life. For example, treat your wetsuit to the occasional wash and store it properly when not in use. Rinse your goggles and costume after use, and hang them to dry.

KIT FOR USE IN THE WATER

There's more to costumes, goggles and swim caps than you might think.

 ## Swimming Costumes for Women

While I'm happy to share my opinions on most things related to outdoor swimming, I am not qualified to offer advice on women's swimming costumes. Instead, I turned for help to Rosie Cook, the founder and CEO of Deakin and Blue, a women's swimwear brand. Here's what she says:

For lots of women even the thought of putting on swimwear is daunting. In fact, body image concerns have driven over 500,000 women to give up swimming in the last 10 years and one in two mums to stop taking their child to learn to swim. These statistics are alarming, but I think most of us can empathise with them: wearing swimwear is as near to naked as we might get in public and swimwear that is ill-fitting or not up to the job can make us feel exposed and self-conscious.

What to consider when picking your swimwear

First and most important is the type of swimming you plan to do, how often, at what temperature and in what sort of water, as this will inform the choice of fabric, features and coverage to look for in your swimsuit or bikini.

Swimmers who are venturing year round into outdoor swim spots will want to look for lined suits or, even better, bonded fabrics, which behave more like neoprene, offering additional warmth for cold swims.

Cold water swimmers and those staying in for longer periods may also look for swimsuits or bikinis with long sleeves for additional coverage.

If you're swimming in the ocean, you'll want to make sure the fabric chosen is resistant to salt water and, wherever you're swimming, a fabric that offers UV protection is critical (year round).

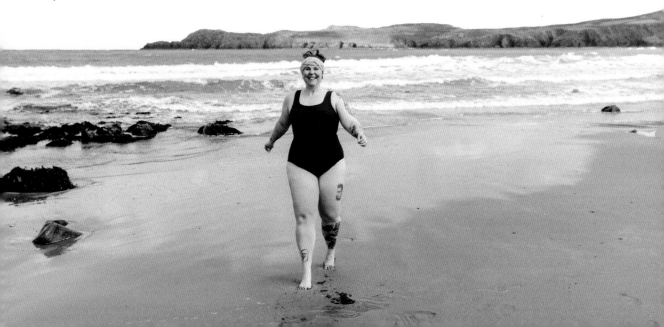

Is it waveproof?

Some outdoor swimmers prefer to swim in a one-piece for the additional coverage (read: warmth) whereas others talk about the ease of lakeside changing in a two piece. Whichever you pick, ease of getting the garment off when you're cold and wet post swim is important – look for zips or clasps for easy changing and stretchy fabrics. If you are going for a bikini, high-waisted bottoms offer additional coverage and are often more waveproof than lower-cut styles (because who wants to go looking for their bikini bottoms in the depths after plunging through the surf?). If you plan to wear a wetsuit on top of your swimwear, make sure you opt for styles that have soft seams so you don't get any unwanted chafing – underarm is the key spot for this.

Does it make you feel comfortable and confident?

It's also important to consider your personal comfort and preferences. Swimwear fit is critical to feeling comfortable and confident in the water. Look for brands that consider bust size as well as dress size to ensure your swimsuit or bikini is truly tailored to your body shape. Swimwear designed for different body shapes doesn't just give proper bust support and shape, but also helps ensure you are hydrodynamic in the water. If you are particularly big busted and planning to do extensive swimming you may also want to look for high-necked styles that will protect you against water channelling between your breasts. You may want to think about your body length and opt for styles that accommodate a longer or shorter body to avoid straps digging into your shoulders or, perhaps worse, slipping off for the duration of your swim. For religious, cultural or other reasons you may be looking for more modest styles and many brands offer swim leggings, rash vests and more covered pieces for these reasons.

And finally, because a large part of the joy of outdoor swimming is embracing the natural world around us, giving thought to the eco-footprint of your swimwear is a worthwhile activity. Opt for eco-friendly fabrics (many brands make swimwear from regenerated nylon rather than virgin yarns), look for brands that produce locally and in small production runs, and for companies who have a transparent supply chain and sustainability credentials, such as a free-of-charge repair service.

MY STORY

Swimmer turned businesswomen

After struggling to find a swimsuit for my weekly swim, I decided to design my own. I wanted to reinvent swimwear, to develop pieces that are transformational in how they feel, how they move and how they are made, and then make a business out of it. I'm on a mission to help women, whatever their shape or size, feel incredible in their swimwear.

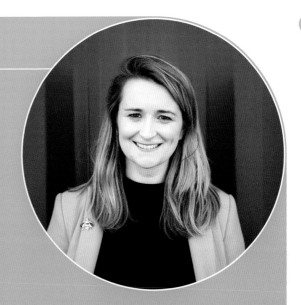

The brand I created, Deakin and Blue, has been worn by Olympic swimmers, professional surfers and head-up breaststrokers alike, as well as being featured in, The Times, Telegraph, Vanity Fair, and more. Every style comes in three curve options to suit a range of body shapes and pieces are available in sizes UK 8-24, AA-HH cup. Every piece is designed and made from ocean waste in East London.

For me, comfort is confidence. When you feel good, you relax and enjoy yourself, so finding swimwear that has been designed to fit your body is critical to enjoying being in the water.

As for my own swimming, you may find me at London Fields Lido or dipping in the Hampstead Ponds.

ROSIE COOK

Other top costume tips from female swimmers

- Bikini bottoms that have a tie cord (like men's trunks) are much more secure (especially when pushing off the wall in a lido) than those without. Side ties don't work as well.
- Bikini tops and costumes that have padding for the bust give support and shape, but they take much longer to dry.
- Costumes that zip up the back are uncomfortable under wetsuits as the double zip digs into your spine (the same is true of costumes that tie as the knot is pressed into your spine by the wetsuit zip).

Swimming Costumes for Men

Swimming costumes for men also present some difficult choices. It's not just a body confidence thing. It's also those not-so-subtle questions from friends and family about whether your choice of swimwear is appropriate. One letter writer to *The Sunday Times* asked for help in persuading her 35-year-old boyfriend to stop wearing Speedos as his 'midriff is not as taut as it was'. Instead of advising that she let her boyfriend make his own swimwear choices and that the size of his midriff was irrelevant, *The Sunday Times'* Style Magazine's agony aunt suggested shaming him into wearing something more appropriate by taking photos of him in his bathers. Horrible advice! And I'm not so sure about the girlfriend either.

Body shaming has no place anywhere and especially not in swimming, where so much of our body is on display. Midriffs, bulging or otherwise, shouldn't be a consideration in your choice of swimwear.

Your choices come down to baggy shorts or skin-hugging briefs, with some variations on both themes. For example, board shorts can be above or below the knee and skin-tight trunks can be mini briefs (as popularised by Speedo), wide-sided briefs, shorts or jammers.

There is no doubt that tight-fitting swimwear is better for swimming. Baggy shorts slow you down and make it harder to swim in a nice horizontal, streamlined

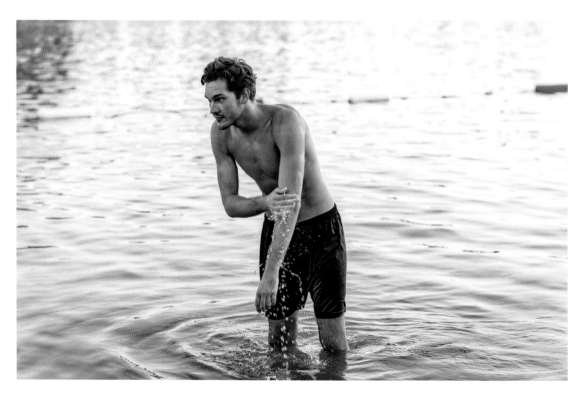

position, and below-the-knee ones are worse. They are also uncomfortable when wet. However, if you feel self-conscious in a skin-tight costume and speed isn't an issue, then wear shorts. If I'm messing about in the water rather than swimming, or combining swimming with another activity such as paddleboarding, I prefer shorts – although I'll usually wear running shorts rather than board shorts. Briefs – sometimes known as 'budgie smugglers' for good reason – can be too revealing. Do what feels right for you.

The only thing to check if you're doing a non-wetsuit swimming event is if they have rules dictating what type of costume you can wear. For example, the British Long Distance Swimming Association (BLDSA) says that your swimming costume shouldn't cover your thighs.

If you're swimming in a wetsuit, baggy shorts will crumple up inside and be uncomfortable. You're better off wearing tight-fitting jammers or briefs, a tri suit, or nothing at all underneath.

As with women's costumes, remember to check the environmental and sustainability credentials of your swimwear.

Board shorts or skin-tight options?

	Board shorts	Skin-tight options (briefs or jammers)
Pros	Less revealing Can be worn for other activities	Faster for swimming More comfortable under a wetsuit
Cons	Create drag for swimming Uncomfortable when wet	Revealing

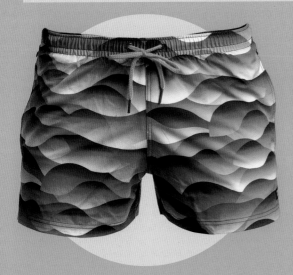

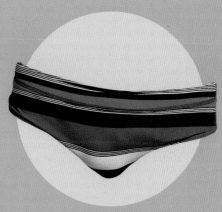

∞ Goggles

I hesitate to recommend goggles. There is such a wide range of options and swimmers often have very strong opinions on which ones are the best. I'm lucky that I can use a wide range of goggles, but I know some people struggle to find any that are comfortable and don't leak. However, most people will find a pair they like, so don't despair if you don't get on with the first couple you try.

While some goggles, are marketed as open water goggles, if you've got a pair you're happy with swimming in the pool, they will be fine in open water too. However, the demands on your goggles will be greater when swimming outside. For example, waves can dislodge poorly fitting goggles. You tend to look up and around more when swimming outside, so clarity and width of vision may be more important, especially if you're racing and need to spot turn markers and the finish line. Lighting varies more outside, so you may want two pairs: a clear pair for overcast days and tinted or polarised lenses for bright sunlight.

Or, if you've got the budget, there are goggles with photochromic lenses. Most goggles offer UV protection, but that's worth checking if you're going to swim outside often.

That said, the most important criteria for goggles are comfort and being leak free. This depends, often, as much on how you fit and adjust them as the brand or style. See page 116 for some tips on wearing goggles.

∞ Racing/performance goggles

Low-profile goggles with relatively small lenses are popular with competitive pool swimmers. They fit securely in your eye socket and most have adjustable nose pieces to suit different face shapes. If these are what you've grown up with and are used to, you may be perfectly happy wearing them in open water. Many of the elite swimmers on the international marathon swimming circuit wear this type of goggles.

Pros: Sleek, fast and look cool. Versatile.

Cons: Narrower field of vision than some other goggles. Less protection for your eyes if you get hit in the face.

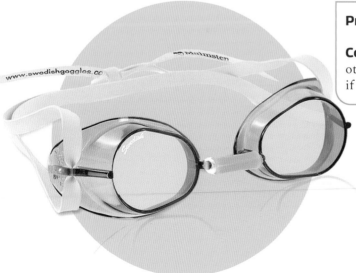

www.swedishgoggles.co

Open water goggles

Designed for swimming outdoors, these have a larger lens than racing goggles. The lens is held in a gasket that sits on the bone around the eye socket rather than within it. Lenses are often curved for a wider field of vision and there are a range of lens types, from clear to tinted, mirrored, polarised and photochromic. Some brands have mechanisms for easy tightening while wearing.

Pros: Good eye protection and clear, wide-angle vision.

Cons: Fixed nose piece doesn't fit all face types.

Mask-style goggles

Large goggles that sit on your eyebrows and cheek bones and leave plenty of clearance for your eyes, eye lashes and (I'm told) mascara. The extra coverage of your face provides additional protection against the cold and vision is unimpeded. For outdoor swimming, it's usually better to use the type of mask that leaves your nose free rather than the scuba-style ones that enclose it.

Pros: Clear vision and comfort (for some people anyway).

Cons: High profile increases chance of being knocked off.

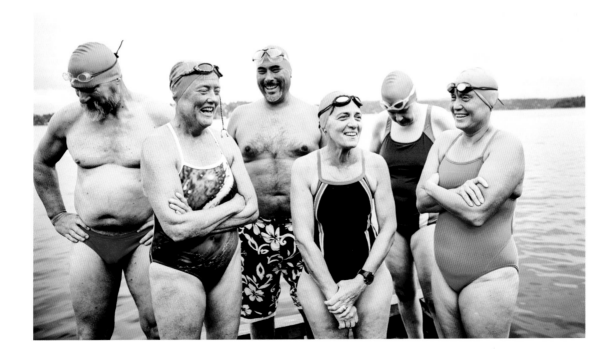

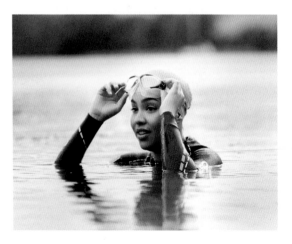

Stop the fog

Nobody likes foggy goggles. But how do you stop them misting up? Most goggles have an anti-fog coating. For new goggles, the best option is usually to put them on dry and keep them dry while you swim. The anti-fog coating can be refreshed with anti-fog sprays.

Goggle manufacturers recommend not touching the lenses, because you can damage the anti-fog coating and greasy fingerprints attract fog. However, once the original anti-fog has stopped working, I find the best way to keep goggles clear is to smear a tiny drop of shampoo around the lenses and then rinse in cold water. Ideally, use a shampoo that won't sting your eyes and make sure you rinse the goggles properly. Spit is an alternative, but it's a bit yuck and I don't find it as effective.

If you find your goggles have misted up in the middle of a swim, a quick rinse will often clear them. You don't need to take them off for this. Lift the seal gently off your face and lower your head into the water, then let the water out again (but don't do this if you're wearing contact lenses – see opposite page for why). If fogging continues, you can leave a few drops of water inside the goggles as you swim (again, this isn't a good idea if you wear contact lenses). As this sloshes around, it clears the fog. However, if you leave too much in, it defeats the purpose of goggles.

Goggle options for glasses wearers

If, like me, you wear glasses, then you have a few options. You can wear normal goggles and muddle through with your fuzzy vision, which may be fine if your prescription isn't that strong; you can buy off-the-shelf prescription goggles for approximate correction; you can buy goggles or masks into which you insert custom prescription lenses; or you can wear contact lenses under regular goggles.

Bear in mind that opticians warn against the contact lens option due to the risk of acanthamoeba infection, which can result in permanent visual loss. Acanthamoeba is a waterborne microbe that's all around us, but the risks of infection go up if you wear contact lenses while swimming. If you still choose to wear contact lenses under goggles (I do sometimes for events), try to keep all water out of your goggles and remove the contact lenses immediately after you finish swimming. This means you will probably need to pack your glasses to put on once you're removed your lenses.

Off-the-shelf prescription goggles only correct for distance, not astigmatism. Unless you have a very basic prescription, swimming goggles will not provide the same level of vision as your glasses, but should suffice for swimming.

To calculate the power for your goggles, you need to consider the two aspects of your prescription, sphere (sph) and cylinder (cyl). The first refers to the amount of short- or long-sightedness you have and the second the amount of astigmatism. It is usually written in the form R -3.00 / -0.50 x 180 and then L -3.50 / -1.00 x 2.

You should base the power for your goggles primarily on the first number – how short- or long-sighted you are. If you also have a moderate degree of astigmatism (up to 2.00), incorporate up to half of this to choose the most appropriate power. Most swimming goggles come in 0.50 or 1.00 steps so you may have to select the nearest power.

If you can't find an off-the-shelf pair of goggles that correct your vision sufficiently for swimming, you may need to look at custom lenses or custom inserts.

My personal favourites are Swans Prescription Goggles, but of course there are other brands. I use the same pair both in the pool and outdoors.

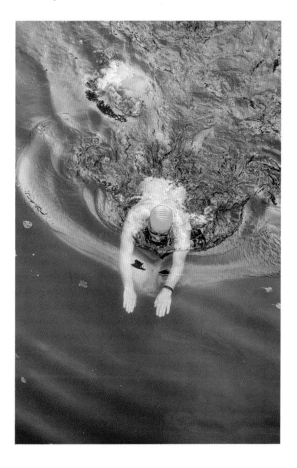

Hi-tech goggles

For many of us, swimming is a refuge from electronic technology and a chance to switch off. However, in recent years, there have been some exciting advances in goggle technology that are worth looking at if you have the interest and budget.

FORM Smart Swim Goggles have developed a pair of goggles with an augmented reality display that beams real-time performance data into your eye as you swim. Originally developed for pool swimmers, it displayed data such as elapsed time and number of lengths swum. A later software update enabled connection to certain GPS sports watches and heart rate monitors for use outdoors. The display can be set to show heart rate, distance swum (based on the watch's GPS readings) and pace. It's quite something to see a green digital display of your speed, apparently suspended in the water just below you, when swimming face down in a murky river. Luckily, the technology is not yet advanced enough to annoy you with Instagram updates while you swim, but I fear it won't be long.

Another product that's recently come on the market is OnCourse Goggles. These were specifically developed for open water swimmers and use sensors to detect the earth's magnetic field. After pointing the goggles in the direction you want to swim, you click a button and go. If you veer off course, lights flash in your eyes indicating the direction you need to swim to get back on course.

No doubt new products are in development and this will be an exciting space to watch.

Swimming without goggles

Goggles aren't essential to enjoy outdoor swimming (unless you need to wear your contact lenses, in which case do always wear goggles). I can think of four situations in which I don't use goggles, as listed below.

1. A spontaneous swim when I don't have kit with me.
2. When the water is extremely cold and I don't want to put my face in so I don't need them.
3. When I'm doing a head-up breaststroke leisure swim.
4. When I'm bodysurfing and goggles would probably get knocked off by the waves.

Otherwise, goggles protect your eyes from the sometimes dirty water and, if you get the opportunity to swim in clear water, to see what's around and beneath you.

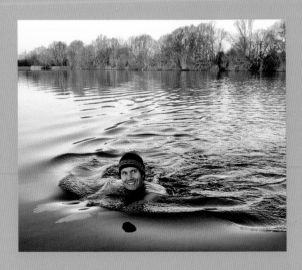

Swimming Caps and Other Head Coverings

Swimming caps and other head coverings serve at least five main purposes for outdoor swimmers:

1. Even the thinnest of swimming caps helps keep some heat in.
2. Caps hold your hair in place.
3. Colourful caps help other water users, swimmers and lifeguards to see you.
4. Swimmers use them to make statements about the races they've done and the clubs or groups they belong to.
5. Fun and swimming hat competitions.

Other uses of swimming caps include holding your goggles in place. I've also seen people use them to carry asthma inhalers. In races, caps are sometimes numbered to help identify swimmers. It's a lot of work for a humble, sometimes optional, and frequently overlooked piece of kit.

The cheapest, thinnest swimming caps are made from latex. These are often the ones you receive at events. Slightly more expensive, but thicker and stronger, are caps made from silicone. Most people I speak to prefer the silicone caps as they tend to fit better, tug on the hair less and are slightly warmer. However, I have met swimmers who prefer the latex ones as they stretch a little more and can accommodate more hair.

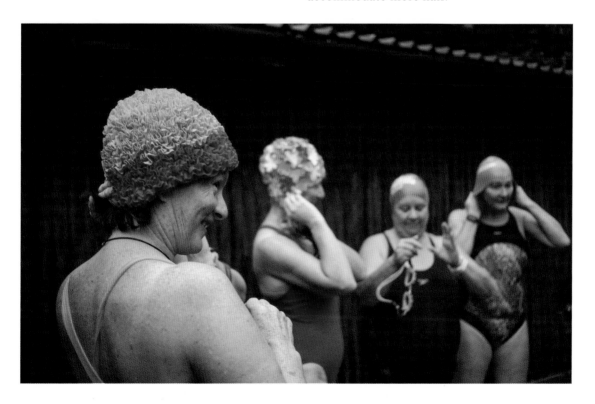

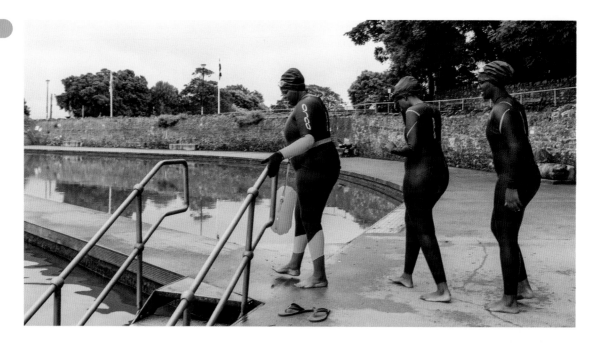

Hats generally come in one size only and stretch with use, but you can also get shaped silicone hats. These are sometimes used by competitive swimmers as it's easier to remove the wrinkles from them and they are therefore more streamlined. Another option is a so-called Bubble Swim Hat. Also made from silicone, this has the same shape, but is a slightly larger size than a regular swimming cap. It also has a textured surface (the bubbles) that's designed to hold in more warmth.

For swimmers with voluminous or afro-type hair, regular-size caps sometimes don't fit. The creators of Soul Cap spotted a gap in the market and set up a business to produce a range of larger caps for swimmers with big hair – or the 'volume-blessed' as they describe it. Their Soul Cap XXL will even cater for waist-length dreadlocks.

For additional warmth, you could try a neoprene swimming cap. These are usually held in place with chin straps that give the sides of your face some protection. If you want full head and neck coverage, you can even get neoprene balaclavas.

Swimming caps in use

- Brightly coloured caps are best for outdoor swimming to help other people see you.
- If you are given a numbered latex cap in a race, but you prefer to wear your own silicone cap, put your cap on first and the latex one on top.
- Use two caps for additional warmth (but note, some events and challenges run under traditional swimming rules only allow the use of a single cap).
- If you use a dark neoprene cap, put a brightly coloured latex or silicone cap on top for visibility.
- Protect your ears by keeping them inside the cap.
- Pull the cap down over your forehead to reduce the chance of it slipping off.
- Take care putting your cap on as they can split. Be careful with sharp nails.
- Dry your cap after use.

Finally, for head-up breaststroke swimming in winter, stylish swimmers wear a bobble hat, usually paired with a brightly coloured swimming costume and neoprene socks and gloves.

Hair care

If you colour your hair or have hair that's easily damaged by exposure to chlorine, salt water or sunlight, then you may want to take extra care of it while swimming. Trichologist and hairstylist (and long-distance swimmer) Julie Hacket recommends using a water-resistant hair mask. As these can make your hair slippery, she wears a Lycra swimming cap underneath her silicone cap to make sure it stays on. To remove the cream from the hair, along with anything else picked up in the water (including chlorine from pool swims), look for a clarifying shampoo that treats damage caused by frequent swimming.

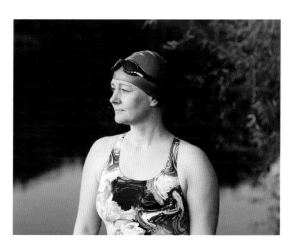

Ear Plugs and Nose Clips

Ear plugs are useful if you are prone to ear infections or swimmer's ear (otitis externa), because they keep the ears dry and out of contact with potentially polluted water. Some swimmers say they also help keep them warmer by stopping cold water coming into the ears. If you frequently swim in cold water, ear plugs may reduce the risk of surfer's ear (exostosis), a condition where the ear canal develops bony growths as a response to repeated cold exposure.

Custom-fitted ear plugs usually provide the best fit. You can also get ear plugs that keep water out, but let sound through. However, when I tried these, I still found they blocked out some sound, so mostly I swim without ear plugs and try to protect my ears with my swimming cap. On the other hand, I know swimmers who always use ear plugs.

As for nose clips, I'm not a fan and I don't see many outdoor swimmers using them. The main reason is that I breathe out through my nose and a clip would obviously prevent that. However, they can be useful in some circumstances, such as swimming underwater on your back (something you'll only likely do in a pool) or perhaps snorkelling if you don't have a snorkelling mask that covers your nose. If you are bothered by water coming up your nose when swimming outside, then by all means see if a nose clip helps. But also practise breathing out through your nose while your face is in the water.

Wetsuits

In my 10 years of publishing *H2Open* and *Outdoor Swimmer* magazine, nothing has been as consistent in stirring debate, inviting controversy and inspiring cutting remarks as the use of wetsuits in outdoor swimming.

It's worth understanding some of the reasons behind this.

Traditionally, swimmers either learned to cope with the water temperature or they didn't swim. Rules for the great swims, such as a recognised English Channel crossing, forbid the use of wetsuits. You can still book and pay for an English Channel swim and do it in a wetsuit, but neither of the two Channel swimming organisations will recognise it as a genuine crossing. Marathon swimming events sanctioned by FINA (the global governing body for swimming) and by national and regional governing bodies also did not allow wetsuits. The same was true for swims organised by the British Long Distance Swimming Association.

As triathlon evolved in the 1970s and 1980s, athletes started using wetsuits for the swim portion of the events and quickly realised that not only did the wetsuit keep you warmer, it also enabled you to swim faster. Businesses soon stepped in to fulfil this new need, developing wetsuits specifically for faster triathlon swimming. Triathlon organisers and governing bodies saw safety benefits: a wetsuit helps you float and a warm swimmer is less likely to become hypothermic on their bike. They introduced rules insisting on wetsuits below certain temperatures. However, because of the speed benefits, the majority of triathletes use them except when the water is too warm and they are forbidden.

Early mass participation open water swimming races were often put on by triathlon organisers and they followed triathlon guidelines rather than traditional swimming rules. Some made wearing wetsuits compulsory.

Naturally, people wondered if they could use wetsuits for traditional swimming events and challenges, setting the scene for years of argument. The current situation is that the traditionalists have defended their flagship challenges and the English Channel and other famous swims must be completed without a wetsuit for official recognition. Elite swimming events, including the 10km (6.2-mile) Olympic marathon swim, have reached a compromise with wetsuits being compulsory below 18°C (64.4°F), optional between 18 and 20°C (64.4–68°F) and banned above 20°C (68°F).

Other traditional organisers continue to encourage non-wetsuit swimming, but have started welcoming wetsuited swimmers and offering prizes in a separate category. The mass participation sector is now mostly wetsuit optional, but some events make wetsuits compulsory. Consequently, you always need to check on an event organiser's policies when you sign up.

These policies have also spilled over into commercial venues. Most allow you to choose whether or not to wear a wetsuit. I don't know of any that don't allow them. Some insist you wear one. However, if you're swimming for your own pleasure and are not ever going to take part in an event, then it's your choice.

Choosing a wetsuit

You can spend a lot of money on a wetsuit. It's therefore worth doing your research and making the right choice. For the occasional wild swimming dip, you can get away with a cheap, general-purpose wetsuit. However, if you want to swim, you will be more comfortable in a wetsuit designed for swimming or triathlon.

For my first open water triathlon, in 1989, I swam in an old sleeveless wetsuit I'd had for kayaking. I'd have been better off without it. Water flooded in under my arms and it ballooned around my waist. It was like trying to swim while dragging a parachute. The swim took me twice as long as it should have done and completely exhausted me. Obviously, I should have tested it before trying to race in it.

Whatever wetsuit you choose, it must fit well. Too tight and it will constrict your movement and breathing. Too loose and water will slosh in, negating the warmth benefits and making it harder to swim. Study the manufacturer's size guides before buying and don't assume that a size you previously had with one brand will be the same with another. The wetsuit should feel tight when you first put it on, but not so tight that you don't have full range of movement.

Pros of wetsuits:
- Keeps you warmer.
- Helps you float.
- Enables most people to swim faster.
- Allows you to swim in places and events that make wetsuits compulsory.

Cons of wetsuits:
- Additional hassle and faff.
- Can cause sores if it rubs and chafes, especially around the neck.
- You can't feel the water against your skin.
- Most lift your legs too high in the water for comfortable breaststroke swimming.

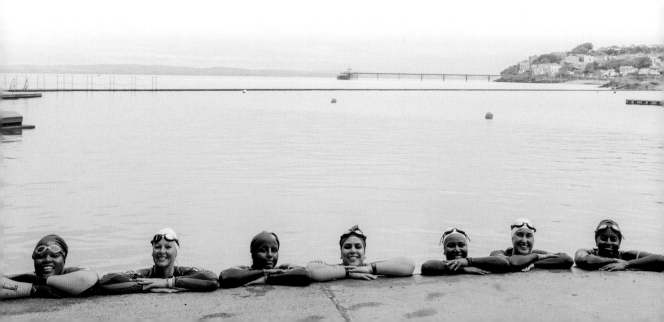

How much should you spend on a wetsuit?

With swimming wetsuits, more money tends to buy you gains in speed. However, in my experience, the difference between the top and bottom of the range is much less than the gains made from going from no wetsuit to an entry level swimming wetsuit. More expensive suits have fewer panels and thinner, more flexible neoprene around the shoulders, resulting in less fatigue while swimming. Swimming in an expensive suit feels more natural than an entry level one. The downside is that expensive suits can be more fragile. Also, because expensive suits are designed for speed rather than warmth, entry level and mid-range wetsuits are often warmer, particularly on the arms and shoulders. There are three main price points:

1. Entry level: £100–250
Great for casual use, wild swimming and the occasional event. Should be robust and warm.

2. Mid-level: £250–400
Improved flexibility around the shoulders and have some speed features, such as special coatings. Good for longer recreational swims and racing, but can be used for any type of swimming.

3. Top end: £400-plus
Everything is designed for speed, including features for rapid removal in a triathlon. Swimming fast in a well-fitting top-end suit is a joy, but these suits are expensive so best reserved for races. They often use thinner materials, especially on the arms, which can be uncomfortable in cold water.

Swimming breaststroke in a wetsuit

Since the evolution of the swimming wetsuit was driven by triathlon, nearly every suit on the market is designed for front crawl. Not only that: they are designed to help runners and cyclists swim faster. Many triathletes come to swimming as adults and often have poor body position while swimming, with their legs too low in the water. Wetsuits have lots of buoyancy around the hips and legs to bring the legs closer to the surface for more streamlined swimming, which is the main reason wetsuits help you swim faster front crawl. The problem is, this isn't a good body position for breaststroke, making it feel awkward and putting strain on your back. Some people say it lifts their legs so high that they kick the air.

With outdoor swimming separate from triathlon becoming more popular, brands have responded by introducing breaststroke wetsuits. At the time of writing, these were so new I hadn't had a chance to try one, but they might be worth considering if you prefer swimming breaststroke. Another option might be to try a swimrun wetsuit as these also have less buoyancy around the legs.

Tow Floats

Tow floats solve one of swimmers' biggest problems when swimming in open water: how to be visible to other water users. Handily, some models solve another problem for swimmers: how to carry your clothes and keep them dry. And while not designed to be life-saving devices, they are great to hang on to if you get cramp, or want to stop for a rest and chat. Some events and venues now make the use of tow floats compulsory, so it's worth checking when you sign up.

A tow float has three parts:

1. A waist strap.
2. A line connecting the strap to the float.
3. The float itself.

Adjust the waist strap so it's tight enough not to slip over your hips, but loose enough so you can slide it around. Some models have a line you can adjust in length. In others, it's fixed. I like the float to be above my knees. If it's too far back, I keep kicking it.

A lightweight tow float is barely noticeable while swimming in calm conditions. In wind and waves, you sometimes feel a gentle tug on your waist as the float is pulled about. Occasionally, with a strong tailwind, the float might be blown along faster than you can swim, and you may catch it with your hand or get the strap looped around your shoulder. It's rare. I wouldn't worry about it. And if it happens, untangle yourself calmly and keep swimming.

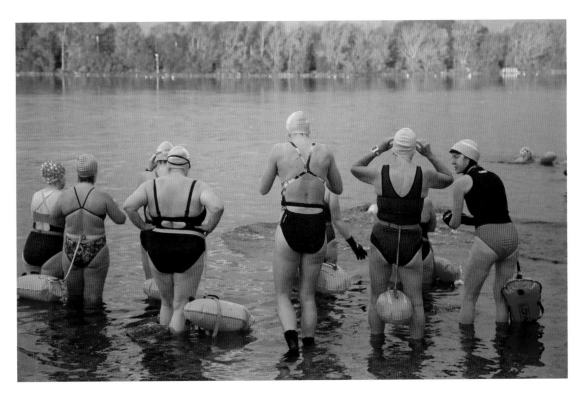

You may notice a slight drag from heavier tow floats or if you've packed one full of clothes. This won't spoil a recreational swim, but if you're racing and every second counts, go for a simple, bag-free float.

For night swimming, attach a waterproof light to the outside of the tow float for additional visibility. Alternatively, if you have a float with a waterproof bag, put a bicycle light inside for a magical glowing float.

It's worth spending some time browsing before buying your first tow float and thinking through what you will use it for. New options and styles appear frequently. If you just want something for your car keys and wallet, a float with a small waterproof pouch will be fine. If you want to carry your phone and have it accessible for taking photos, go for one with an external pocket (but make sure your phone is securely fastened to the float). Other options include floats to carry bottles and snacks through to ones with bags big enough to carry a complete change of clothes. Remember, you need to close the bags properly to keep your kit dry.

Variations on the tow float theme

There are a couple of other innovations that are worth looking at, depending on the type of swimming you want to do. For the adventurous, there's RuckRaft, a towable floating raft big enough for all your camping gear while on the water, but that packs up small enough to carry in your rucksack for hiking to your next swim spot. I spoke to one swimmer who uses one to carry her crutches while swimming so she always has them handy.

Another device that might come in handy – perhaps for coaches looking after multiple people in the water, or in situations where a tow float is awkward, such as surf or in some races – is an emergency inflatable float. I've seen a couple of options for this. The first, called Tekrapod, sits between you shoulder blades in a mini, streamlined rucksack. The other, from Restube, you carry in a pouch on a strap around your waist. Both are inflated in seconds from a CO_2 gas canister that you release with a sharp tug on a pull cord. As with all kit, there are always innovations and different brands, so it's worth exploring all the current options.

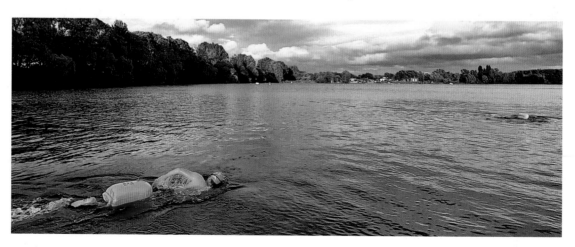

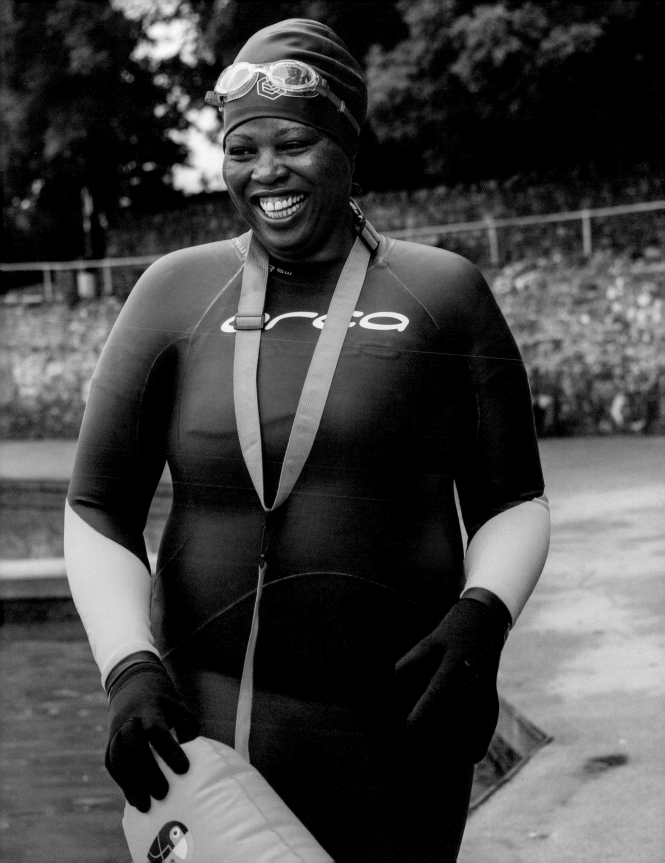

Neoprene Accessories

Sometimes your hands and feet need a little extra protection, either from the cold or sharp surfaces. Neoprene gloves and socks or booties are worth considering, especially if you suffer from Raynaud's. At the beach, foot protection reduces the risk of weever fish and stingray stings.

The downside of both socks and gloves is that you lose your connection with the water and this makes swimming feel clumsy. Also, if you have poorly fitting accessories, they will fill with water. Not only will they then not keep you so warm, but the extra weight makes it even harder to swim. Luckily, you can now buy swimming-specific neoprene accessories that minimise (but don't eliminate) these issues. With both socks and gloves, the thicker the neoprene, the more protection you get

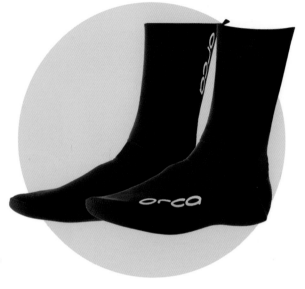

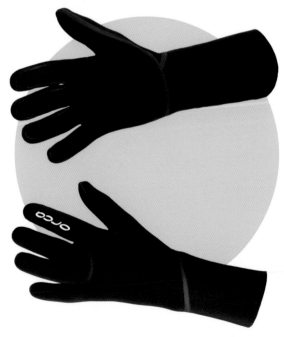

from the cold, but thicker material also makes you feel more awkward while swimming.

In the winter, you often see the curious sight of swimmers in bathing costumes while wearing neoprene socks and gloves. This might strike you as a little odd but it makes sense. In cold water, especially below about 5°C (41°F), hands and feet can become extremely painful, while water on the body just feels cold. The layer of neoprene on your hands and feet takes away the pain and allows you to enjoy the swim more. Another advantage is that when you finish the swim, you can use your hands. I've done swims without gloves when my fingers got so cold I was unable to undo the clip of my tow float or the lace of my trunks.

You might need to try a few different brands and sizes to find the ones that fit and suit you best.

Neoprene socks and gloves in use

If using socks and gloves while wearing a wetsuit, you can usually keep water out by pulling the sleeves of the wetsuit over the cuffs or the other way around. Experiment to see which method works for you. When using them without a wetsuit, you may need to be creative in keeping the water out. I've seen, for example, people using Velcro straps around their wrists.

For winter swimming, it's important to dry off and dress quickly, and gloves may hinder this. In some cases, it may be better to put a changing robe on first, and then remove your gloves. Dress your top half before taking off your neoprene socks.

If you're starting outdoor swimming in the summer, I wouldn't rush into buying neoprene gloves or socks, unless you need foot protection because of where you swim. Your hands and feet may feel painfully cold when you first get in – and I find they can feel worse if you're wearing a wetsuit, as if all the cold is concentrated in your extremities – but you should get used to it within a few minutes. You will have a better swimming experience without gloves or socks. Moving through autumn and winter, I would also recommend staying glove free as long as you can. Both your hands and feet adapt, to an extent, as temperatures drop.

Other Useful In-water Accessories

 ### Sports watches

If you want a rough estimate of how far you've swum in open water, a GPS sports watch is a reasonable guide. However, they don't work under water. If you're swimming front crawl, your arm is usually out of the water long enough and often enough for distance measurement to work. Even so, when I swim with friends, there is sometimes up to 20 per cent difference in the distances we measure. For better distance measurement, you can clip your watch to your tow float so it's permanently above water (double-check it's secure), but

then you lose other metrics such as stroke and heart rate.

In the winter, I always wear a stopwatch to keep track of the time to make sure I don't stay in too long.

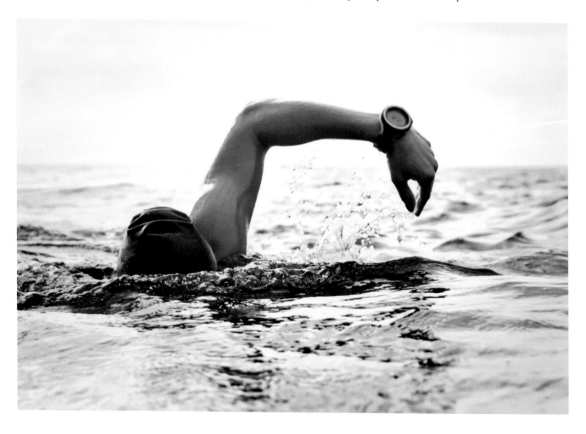 ### Waterproof phone pouch

If you're wild swimming, it's a good idea to have a phone with you in case of emergencies, but carry it in a fully waterproof (and tested) pouch and secure the pouch to your body or tow float. If you have a clear pouch, you can also use your phone to take photos.

I recently lost a phone in a river when the line I used to attach it around my waist snapped. Check and recheck your kit before swimming.

Waterproof camera

You can get some great photos from the water, but you need the right camera. Action cameras, such as GoPro, work well, but make sure they are properly waterproof before taking them swimming. Some cheaper and older models need to be carried inside a waterproof housing. There are also waterproof cameras that are small enough to slip inside your costume, which makes them easy to swim with, but, again, think through how to keep them secure.

Whistle

A pea-less whistle is useful for attracting attention in emergencies – for example, if a rowing boat is bearing down on you. A few tow floats now have these fitted as standard and you also find them on the zips of some swimrun wetsuits.

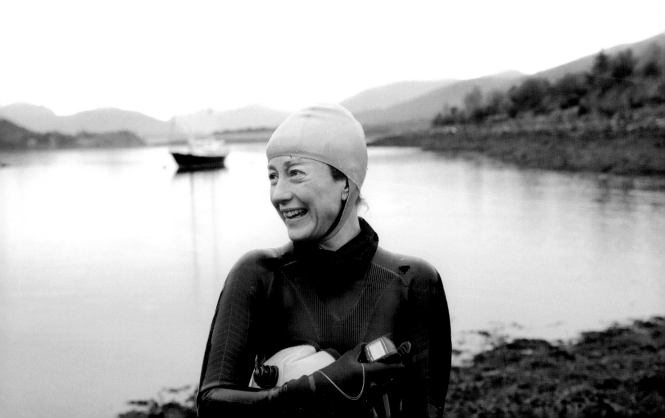

MY STORY

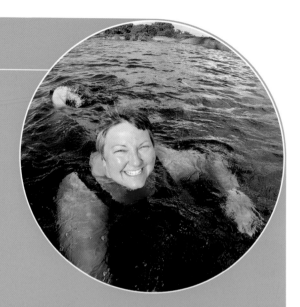

The swimsuit issue: don't tell me I'm brave

It is not unusual to be asked about how I manage to be comfortable being photographed in my swimwear. How can I appear in publications or social media in JUST my swimsuit? Simply asking these questions is a reminder that society, culture and marketing have programmed us to see a female swimming body in a certain way. Telling me I am brave for doing so is just as bad as telling me I don't belong in a swimsuit at my size.

I have been swimming my whole life and spent a decade swimming at events with all kinds of swimmers. From a mile sea swim to marathon distances in rivers or hours of swimming loops in lakes, I completed and succeeded at outdoor swimming. On land, I feel cumbersome and clumsy. In water, I feel graceful, weightless and glide through time. It is never about speed or winning for me. It is about distance and achievement; setting a goal and seeing if it is possible.

I firmly believe the best open water swimmers are those with a strong mind and who swim long and strong strokes. Standing toes on the edge at the start of any event, I often look out of place. Not choosing to wear a wetsuit and standing in just my costume can lead to judgement. Maybe I look naive or unprepared? But often, when in the water, I swim past those who stared or sneered 'helpful' unsolicited advice at the start line. We are all the same in the water. Beneath the surface you can't see what a swimmer's body is like, nor does it matter.

ELLA FOOTE

Biosecurity – stop the spread

One of the joys of wild swimming is exploring different places. Unfortunately, on your travels between sites, you may have uninvited and unwanted hitch-hikers – invasive, non-native species that can spread rapidly and devastate native species. These can be in the form of viable plant fragments, larvae or eggs.

The GB Non-native Species Secretariat says invasive plants include Australian swamp-stonecrop, floating pennywort, water primrose and parrot's feather. Invasive invertebrates include zebra mussels, quagga mussels, killer shrimps and signal crayfish. As well as competing with native species, they can spread disease and parasites.

The guidance for swimmers and boaters (or anyone travelling between different watercourses) to help stop the spread is: check, clean, dry.

CHECK

Check your equipment and clothing for live organisms – particularly in areas that are damp or hard to inspect.

CLEAN

Clean and wash all equipment, footwear and clothes thoroughly. Use hot water when possible. If you do come across any organisms, leave them at the water body where you found them.

DRY

Dry all equipment and clothing – some species can live for many days in moist conditions. Make sure you don't transfer water elsewhere.

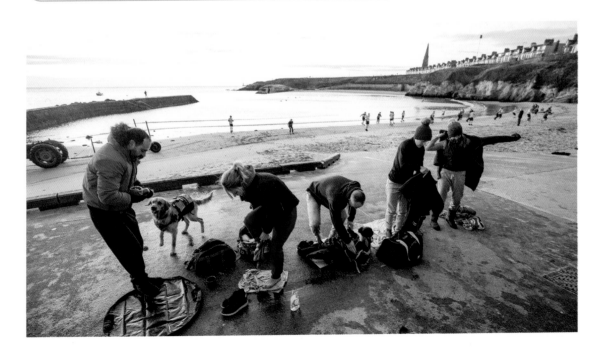

PRE AND POST SWIM

What you use and wear pre and post swim is as important as what you use during your swim, especially in the winter and cooler conditions.

To maximise enjoyment of your swim, you should ensure you are warm before you start and have everything you need to warm up again afterwards. While a spontaneous dip can be fun, only do it when you have enough clothes with you, bearing in mind that you may need extra layers after getting cold. Your regular clothes will mostly be adequate, but if you end up standing around on a chilly beach for a while before or after you swim, you'll be glad to have the additional insulation.

 Changing Robes

These are useful both before and after swimming. The simplest versions are towel robes. More expensive options have a fleecy inner lining and a waterproof shell. They come in a wide range of colours and styles, although stylish they are not. You use these for practical reasons rather than fashion, although they've become so popular in some places they've provoked something of a backlash.

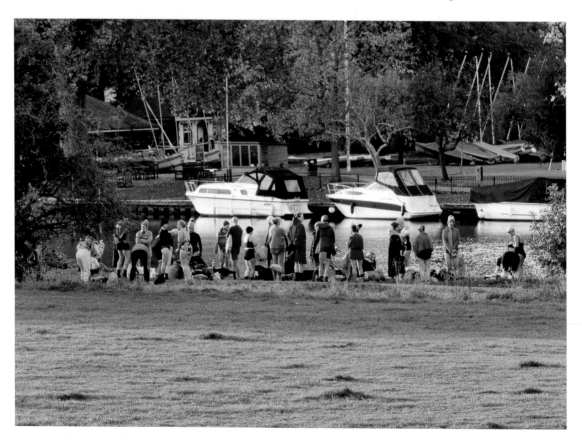

A sign posted at a swimming spot in Ireland in 2020 read: 'No Dryrobes or Dryrobe types' – referring to the brand whose name has become synonymous with changing robes.

I use mine more for keeping warm and warming up than for changing inside, but plenty of swimmers do use them for changing. They are especially handy if you need to hang around in your costume or wetsuit before a swim, as on a cool day it's easy to get cold even in a wetsuit. In winter, after a cold swim, I sometimes put mine on over the top of a coat for extra warmth and I don't care how silly it looks, because it makes a big difference to warming up.

The main downside with the waterproof changing robes (apart from the price) is the bulk. Get a compression sack if you need to pack it down small.

Flip-flops, Sliders and Foam Clogs

Summer or winter, it's good to have something to protect your feet. When it's cold or muddy, I stand on mine while changing, too. If you need to take them into the water with you, pass the lead of your tow float through the straps. They might drag in the water, but it doesn't matter. I've seen a few swimmers using fleece-lined foam clogs in the winter. They look hideous, but I might get some.

Changing Mat

You can buy changing mats that turn into bags. Stand on the mat to change, drop all your wet stuff on to it, then close it up using a drawstring. Alternatively, cut out a piece of old groundsheet or tarpaulin from a tent or similar. When the ground is wet and cold, it makes it more comfortable for changing. Additionally, if it's raining, you can wrap your bag and kit in your changing mat while swimming to keep it dry.

Other useful stuff

- **Towel:** There are lots of choices, including lightweight travel options.
- **Warm clothes:** Easy-to-put-on layers are best. Have at least two more layers in reserve for after your swim than you would wear beforehand.
- **Hat, gloves and thick socks:** It's useful to keep these with you, even in summer, to help with warming up after swimming.
- **Waterproof boots or shoes:** In winter, slip-on options are better in case your fingers are too numb to tie laces.
- **Waterproof bag:** Use this to ensure your kit stays dry.
- **Thermos flask:** For your favourite post-swim warm drink.
- **Hot water bottle:** This keeps your clothes warm while you're swimming and is useful for comfort after your swim, but don't hold it directly against your skin.
- **Large shopping bag:** While you can get all sorts of fancy swimming bags, a big bag-for-life is a cheap and practical option. I've seen people standing inside their bags-for-life while changing.

KIT FOR POOL TRAINING

While this is a book about outdoor swimming, many people swim both in swimming pools and in the wild. A pool is a great place to practise swimming in a controlled and warm environment.

If you're looking to improve your technique or do any structured training, then consider heading to the pool – either to swim on your own or to join lessons or a club. For the latter two, your coach or instructor might ask you to do certain drills or exercises, some of which require some specialised kit. Here's a quick glossary so you're familiar with the terms. For proper usage, it's best to get advice from a coach or swimming teacher, since incorrect use can result in injury. *See* p. 150 for more information on how some of them are used to improve front crawl technique.

Indoor kit and its uses

Item	Description	Use
Kickboard	A large, flat float	Kicking drills
Pull buoy	An elongated figure-of-eight-shaped float	Hold between your legs (usually your thighs) to focus on upper body movement
Hand paddles	Shaped bits of plastic you attach to your hands	Technique drills and building strength
Fins or flippers	Swimmers usually use small versions of divers' fins	Kicking drills, speed swimming, strength building
Central snorkel	A snorkel that sits in front of your face rather than at one side	Swimming technique drills
Tempo trainer	A waterproof metronome	Clip to your goggles or under your swim cap for a regular beep to help with pacing or stroke rate

Note: Some pools do not allow the use of kit in public sessions.

WHAT TO DO WITH YOUR OLD KIT

Unfortunately, a lot of kit for swimming is not recyclable or reusable. It is best, therefore, to only buy what you need and to make sure it's sourced as sustainably as possible. Then, look after your kit to get as much use out of it as possible.

Look out for recycling and reuse schemes. For example, one charity used to collect old goggles, clean and disinfect them, and ship them to swimming schools in developing countries. You can also explore ways you can reuse old kit yourself. I've seen bunting made from swimming caps and computer bags made from old wetsuits. You can also cut the legs and sleeves off old wetsuits to make arm or leg warmers, or even insulation for your coffee cup.

It's likely that more reuse and recycling options will become available in the future, so do some research before sending your old stuff to landfill.

CHAPTER 8

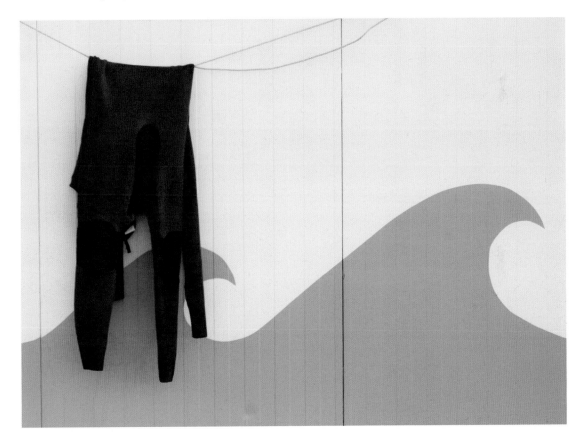

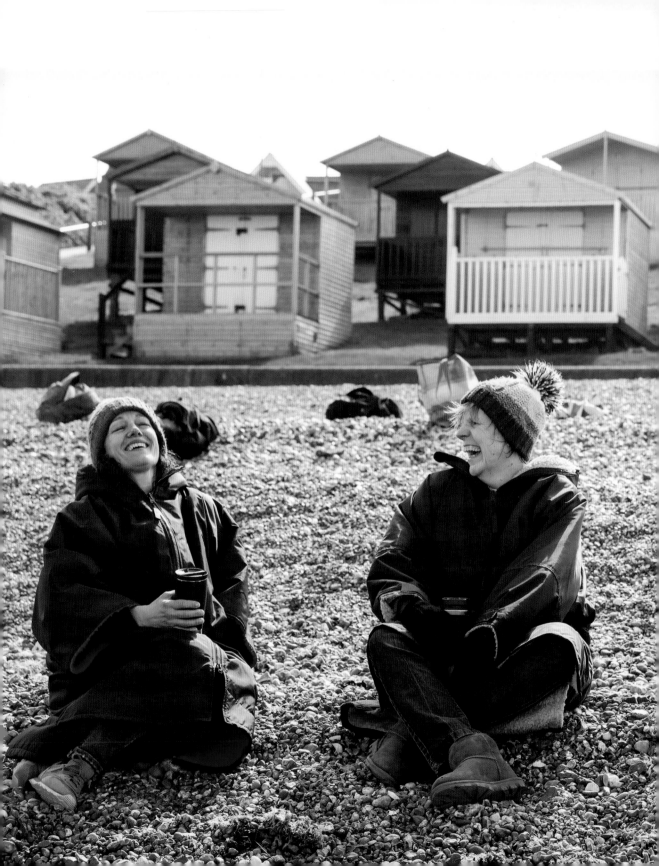

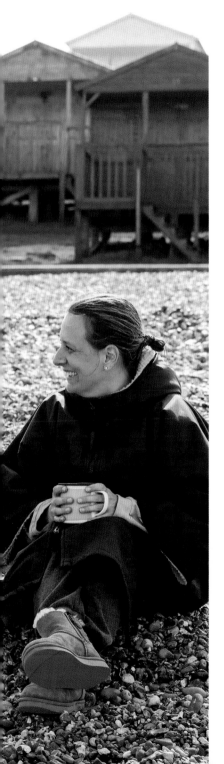

OUTDOOR SWIMMING FOR HEALTH AND WELL-BEING

Swimming outdoors, and especially swimming in cooler water, has a long association with improving and supporting our health and well-being. In this chapter, we look at some of the science behind this and how you can tap into the healing power of water.

WHAT SWIMMING DOES TO YOUR BODY AND MIND

Outdoor swimmers have long maintained their activity is good for them. Science is starting to understand why.

Susie Parr's brilliant book, *The Story of Swimming*, refers to a publication from 1581 by Richard Mulcaster (*Positions*) that suggests swimming in cold water can alleviate headaches, dropsies, scabs, scurf, smallpox and leprosies. Parr also references Sir Everard Digby's 1587 *Art of Swimming*, which claimed swimming could purge poisonous humours and drive away contagious diseases, thereby extending life.

Numerous books and anecdotes now attest to the health and well-being benefits of outdoor swimming. Dr Heather Massey, a researcher at the University of Portsmouth, says cold water swimming has been linked to reductions in blood pressure, pain, menopause symptoms, migraines and colds (*see* Further reading and references on pp. 202–203 for more on this). It's a strongly held belief in swimming circles that regular dips, especially in cold water, boost your immune system. However, while Massey says there are plausible reasons why swimmers might see these benefits, research still needs to be done

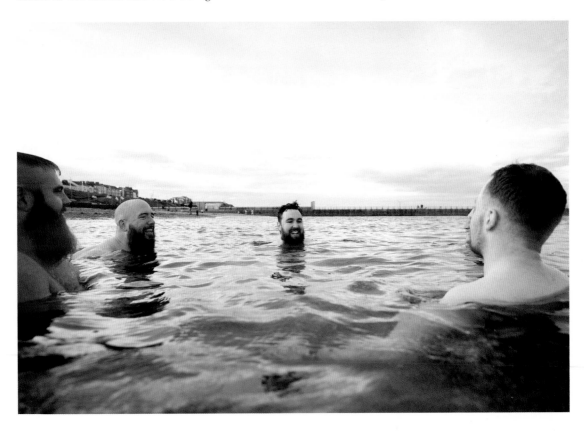

to untangle exactly what is going on from a physiological perspective.

We do know, however, that cold water immersion results in a surge in hormones such as dopamine, serotonin and beta-endorphins, which are associated with improved mood. Another hypothesis suggests that regular exposure to cool water promotes adaptations to stress that may help you cope better with the ups and downs of daily life. It's as if the simple action of provoking a stress response by immersing yourself in cool water trains you to handle stress better in general. Outdoor swimming may make you more resilient.

On a related note, there is now widespread evidence that connecting with nature, and with green and blue spaces, does us good. For example, in her book, *Losing Eden*, Lucy Jones says our well-being depends on nature and this has been known for centuries, and that there is now increasing scientific evidence supporting this. And how could you connect better with nature than by submerging yourself in a pond, lake or river?

There's more: the NHS suggests five evidence-based steps to mental well-being, helping us feel positive and getting the most out of life. The first is 'connect with other people'. Swimmers often spend more time over coffee, cake and a chat than they do in the water, bonding over the shared positive experience of the water.

We're also encouraged to be physically active. Luckily, according to the mental health charity Mind, exercise doesn't need to be intense to achieve mental wellness benefits. A relaxing, low-effort swim is perfect. Equally, if you enjoy the burn of higher-intensity activity, swimming can give you that, too.

Another recommendation is to learn new skills. Outdoor swimming fits the bill for this, too. Not only does it give you the opportunity to work on physical and co-ordination skills, but you also learn about a wide range of topics connected to the activity – this book is just the start. I've been swimming all my life and I still work on my swimming skills and frequently learn new things.

Giving to others is a powerful way to help us look after our mental well-being and that's easy to do in swimming. Thousands of people in the world of outdoor swimming give their time to support and encourage others. The example that most prominently springs to my mind is Freda Streeter, who spent more than 30 years coaching and cajoling trainee English Channel swimmers. Every weekend, from May through to September, Freda travelled to Dover and freely shared her Channel swimming wisdom.

As a new swimmer, you might think you don't have anything to give, but that's not true. You can always bring cake, or you may be the person who has the spare pair of goggles or towel to lend a fellow swimmer.

If you see some rubbish lying around on the ground at your swim spot, pick it up and give the next swimmer a cleaner place to swim. And even after just one outdoor swim, you have valuable experience you can share with someone who is doing their first swim. Everyone has something they can give.

Finally, we're urged to pay attention to the present moment. Well, not much catches your attention like stepping into cold water. And safety demands you monitor your surroundings.

MY STORY

The swim that changed everything

My first swim with MHS Mental Health Swims (see opposite) changed everything. The group welcomed me with warm smiles. The atmosphere was upbeat and positive. The moment I submerged myself in cold water and surrendered to the sea, something incredible happened. My thoughts, fears, anxieties and negative beliefs evaporated, and my mind was silenced. I felt a peace I'd been desperate for. And when I looked around, I saw that others felt the same.

Afterwards, I had a glow that lasted for hours and it became something I needed to do again and again! I felt so passionately about the positive effect it had on my well-being, I wanted to share it with others who might also benefit.

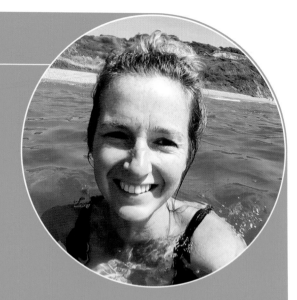

Feeling more alive and inspired than I had in years, I quit my job in finance and I'm now retraining as an outdoor life coach. Alongside this, I regularly write articles and guides with a focus on well-being in nature.

RACHAEL BOUGHTON

For people living with a mental illness diagnosis or mental health challenges, outdoor swimming can be a massive help. The *British Medical Journal* (BMJ) has published a case study documenting how one patient reduced and then ceased their medication after they became a regular outdoor swimmer (*see* Further reading and references on pp. 202–203 for more on this). Scientists describe possible physiological mechanisms through which cold water immersion could boost mood and alleviate some mental health symptoms. One hypothesis is that cold water adaption could reduce the magnitude of pro-inflammatory triggers. This is beneficial because inflammation is linked to a range of conditions, including type-2 diabetes, Alzheimer's and depression.

CASE STUDY
MENTAL HEALTH SWIMS: CELEBRATING THE HEALING POWER OF COMMUNITY AND COLD WATER

If you are considering taking up outdoor swimming for health reasons, Mental Health Swims (MHS) could be a good place to start. After discovering the healing power of outdoor swimming for her own mental health illness, Rachel Ashe created MHS, a not-for-profit organisation that celebrates the healing power of community and cold water. Within two years, she had set up a network of 'Swim Hosts', who host outdoor swims (or dips) at locations around the UK, where everyone is welcome. The swims take place at least once per month, throughout the year.

Rachel champions kindness as an antidote to mental health stigma and this feeds into the operations of MHS, which runs as a peer support community.

At an MHS swim, you should expect that your Swim Host has received training in basic cold water safety, mental health awareness in sport and risk assessment. Swim Hosts aim to provide a welcoming, safe swimming experience. Many also have a lived experience of mental health illnesses. However, while some are qualified lifeguards and outdoor swimming coaches, this is not a requirement.

Therefore, while you should feel safe and welcome, all participants in MHS must take responsibility for their own safety.

An MHS swim works as follows: swim Hosts use the app what3words to share meeting places for swims, where they fly a pink pirate flag to identify themselves. After reading out the MHS disclaimer, the Swim Host counts swimmers into the water. Swimmers are encouraged to stay within their depth and to look out for each other. They refer to 'dips not distance'. The point is a shared experience of the water, not an endurance challenge. Following the swim, participants are encouraged to take part in a 10-minute litter pick.

One of Rachel's ambitions is for MHS to be offered by GPs through social prescribing. However, while she values the huge positive impact outdoor swimming has on our mental health, she says it is not a cure-all. Although there are stories from people who have been able to give up their medication after taking up outdoor swimming, that is not true for everyone. In addition, MHS cannot replace therapy or professional treatment.

Living with a mental health illness and accessing outdoor swimming

Rachel Ashe, founder of Mental Health Swims, shares her top tips for starting and sticking to an outdoor swimming habit for people living with mental health issues:

It's really hard living with a mental illness. Recovery takes a long time and a lot of commitment. Swimming is a possible exception. The impact is instant. There is something empowering about getting outside in winter and swimming. Many swimming groups and all Mental Health Swims groups are welcoming environments regardless of your swimming ability, fitness level and body shape. If you're living with a mental health challenge and want to try outdoor swimming, consider the following:

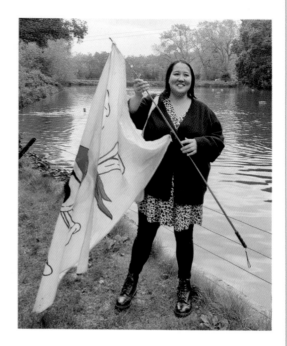

1. Put your clothes in a pile next to your bed. By standing on them when you get out of bed you will be prompted to put them on.
2. Wear your swimsuit under your clothes to make it as easy as possible. It's harder to change your mind about going for a swim if you are still wearing it five hours later (I know this from experience).
3. Pack your bag the night before and have it ready by the front door. Minimise all the reasons for giving up.
4. Find yourself a theme tune to blast out or sing in your head (my current song is 'Castles' by Freya Ridings).
5. Get your breakfast ready the night before (overnight oats or a sandwich are my favourites). I am a firm believer that everything is easier with tasty food.

6. Put Post-it notes with encouraging messages around your home. Make sure they are in all the places you'll see them while getting ready (on the back of the bathroom door, on the mirror, on the kettle).
7. If you have a negative internal monologue, try adopting a kinder one to counter your own (mine is an enthusiastic granny who calls me 'pet').
8. Look up www.mentalhealthswims. co.uk and find your local dip. We welcome and encourage everyone, no matter how they are feeling. We can't wait to meet you! Contact the organiser in advance if you are unsure about anything.

MY STORY

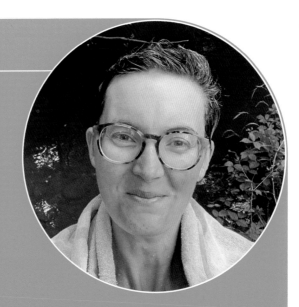

Sharing the joy

As a well-being coach and an avid outdoor swimmer, the concept of Mental Health Swims really resonates with me. I have lived with mental health challenges and outdoor swimming is a real tonic for many reasons. I was initially nervous about becoming a Swim Host because of the potential drain on my energy and impact on my own well-being, but I love that I can share the joy of outdoor swimming.

I discovered wild swimming when I returned from working in Australia. I was lonely and struggling to connect with people. I first ventured to a local swimming venue, where I swam laps in my wetsuit, which was lovely.

However, I didn't feel I'd arrived and connected until I joined a group of wild swimmers and bonded over skinny dipping, cake and tea.

KATIE MACLEOD PETERS

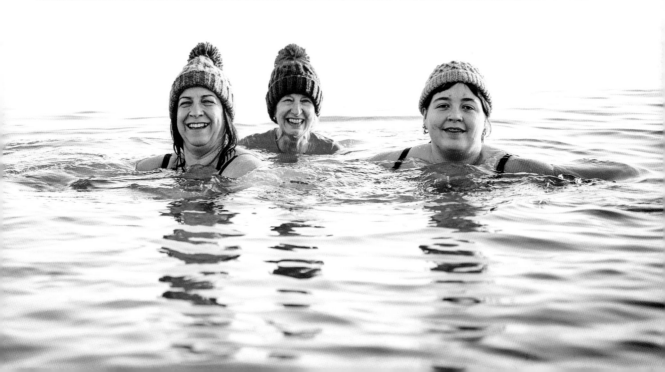

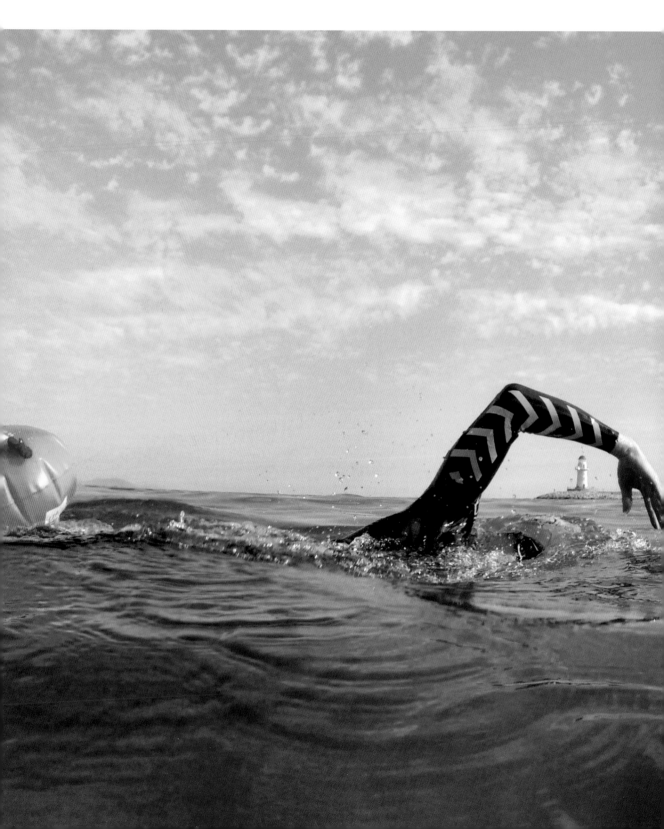

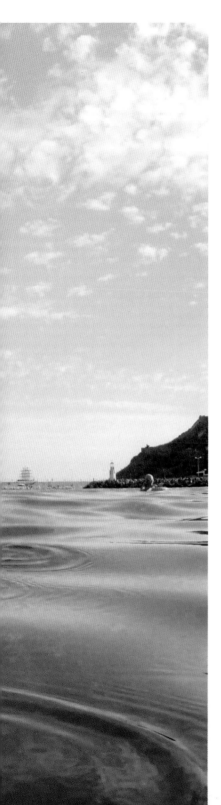

CHAPTER 9

BECOMING A STRONGER SWIMMER

Swimming training and technique are huge topics and the subject of many excellent books (*see* Further reading and references on pp. 202–203 for some suggestions if you want to dive deeper into this). This introduction will help you get started for your first event.

SWIM FURTHER AND FASTER

It's entirely acceptable to do all of your outdoor swimming at a gentle, unhurried pace. Learning to swim further and faster, perhaps for a race or to try a long-distance swimming challenge, is optional, but can be a lot of fun.

In brief, if that is your goal, there are five main components to swimming further and faster in open water:

1. Your swimming technique.
2. Your overall physical fitness and your swim-specific fitness.
3. Your ability to cope with the conditions.
4. Your open water skills.
5. Your mental preparation.

Ideally, you should spend time on the attributes listed above if you want to swim faster and further. Of course, if you're happy with your swimming abilities and enjoy your swims, there is no need to train. On the other hand, many people enjoy the training and skills development process. I love the occasional tough training session, working against the clock, feeling strong and afterwards being tired but satisfied. Luckily, outdoor swimming gives you all the options.

A useful first step is to think through what you enjoy about outdoor swimming and what you want from it – and I hope other parts of this book have given you some ideas for this. Any training you do should either be enjoyable in its own right or help you achieve something you want, and preferably both. Don't 'train' because you think you ought to. You can get all the benefits of outdoor swimming from just doing it. Simply swimming more often will support your fitness and your well-being.

Whatever type of swimmer you are, there is a good chance you will enjoy learning more about swimming technique, practising how to swim more efficiently, becoming more competent in open water, and building your swimming fitness in a systematic and measurable way. At the very least, read this section and experiment with some of the ideas. If it's not for you, there's no harm done and you can continue enjoying swimming as you always have done.

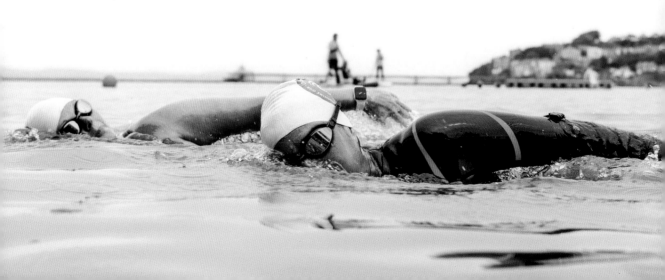

SWIMMING TECHNIQUE

Because swim speed is so dependent on technique, there are opportunities to get faster, whatever age you start.

Whatever stroke you swim, improving your technique is usually the quickest way to improving your speed and efficiency. What's more, swimming with good technique will help reduce your risk of injury. The process to go through is:

1. Understand what good technique looks like.
2. Assess your current technique and identify the gaps between how you swim now and how you would like to swim.
3. Work out what you need to do to improve.
4. Practise.

In reality, it's a lifelong journey. Even swimmers who have seemingly perfect technique will be looking for further refinements or they will regularly do drills and exercises to maintain their form. If you constantly train for fitness and don't pay heed to technique, poor habits can creep in. When you try to make changes to one part of your stroke, you may affect what's happening to a different part of your body. If your neck and shoulders stiffen up from being hunched over a desk all day, it will impact your swimming technique.

The most efficient way to improve your swimming technique is through one-to-one lessons with a skilled coach. While this is expensive, the detailed feedback you'll receive will help you make improvements rapidly. A lot of coaches use video analysis, either in a regular pool or in an endless pool (a type of pool where you swim against a current – a bit like a treadmill for swimmers). Video is a brilliant tool for showing you what you actually do and look like while swimming. It can be quite different to what you think and feel yourself doing.

Swimming involves a complex sequence of movements and it's not possible to focus on all of them at the same time. While you're thinking about your hands, your feet will be doing their own thing. A video recording will help you understand how the various movement patterns link together.

If one-to-one lessons aren't an option, look for group swimming technique classes or courses, which can be a cheaper and more social option. Failing that, get a friend to observe you swimming and give you feedback based on your instructions of what you want them to look for. If you're in an environment where photography is allowed, ask them to film you so you can do your own analysis.

While you can work on swimming technique in open water, it is often easier in a pool, where the water is clear and you don't need to worry about keeping warm. Also, watch videos of top swimmers (there are thousands on YouTube) to see how they swim.

Front crawl is the stroke most people want to improve, so let's review some of the basics for that here. Technical descriptions for the other three recognised competitive strokes (butterfly, backstroke and breaststroke) are beyond the scope of this book but please *see* Further reading and references on pp. 202–203 for suggestions on where to look if this is something you would like to pursue, or seek the help of a qualified swimming teacher or coach.

Front Crawl Fundamentals

Body position

Fast swimmers are close to horizontal in the water. Their shoulders, hips and feet will all be roughly at water level. With slower swimmers, you often see the legs hanging much lower in the water. This increases resistance and makes it harder to swim fast. It's also why wetsuits help a lot of people swim faster: the extra buoyancy lifts their legs closer to the surface.

However, you can't just force your legs closer to the surface. Kicking harder will help, but only temporarily as kicking is exhausting, so it's not a good solution. Most long-distance swimmers do not kick hard, but their feet stay near the surface. Besides, many novice swimmers have poor kicking mechanics and may increase drag with ineffective leg movements if they try to kick harder.

Sinking legs are often a symptom of faults elsewhere in the stroke, such as lifting your head too high, pressing down with your hands at the front of the stroke, poor breathing habits, a weak core or a combination of these factors. If you can make improvements in those other areas, your body position will improve. If you diagnose sinking legs in your stroke, try to identify the fundamental cause rather than consciously working to lift your legs.

As well as your position along the length of your body, you also need to consider it in the other horizontal plane. Imagine being underwater and watching someone swimming front crawl towards you. Now imagine a red line running through their shoulders. If the swimmer were floating face down, this line would be horizontal. But when they swim, the line rocks from side to side with each arm stroke. Swimmers don't swim flat, they switch from their left to right side with each stroke. The amount of rotation is usually around 30–45 degrees and varies between swimmers.

This rotation is important for several reasons: (1) it helps with breathing, as we'll see opposite; (2) it reduces strain on the shoulders during the recovery phase of the stroke; (3) it helps utilise your *latissimus dorsi* muscles (your lats), which adds strength and power to your swimming. Since knowing how much you are rotating is hard to judge on your own, ask someone to watch you swim and give you feedback. While rotation is good, too much will destabilise your swimming and slow your stroke rate, so don't overdo this.

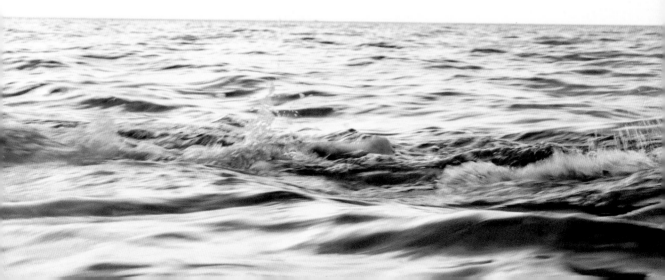

Breathing

Survival instincts push us to get our mouths away from water when breathing in and to hold our breath if our face is in the water. Neither instinct is helpful for efficient swimming. Possible consequences include pushing your legs down and slowing your stroke rate, contributing to feeling breathless or even a sense of panic.

Watch how fast swimmers keep their heads so low it almost looks as if they are breathing under the water. In fact, they find air below the surface level, in the trough created by the bow wave around their head. They then breathe out through their nose and mouth while their face is down. This is a key point to practise. Let the air out while your face is in the water so that you only need to breathe in (not out then in) when your mouth is clear of the water. As you only need to breathe in while your mouth is clear of the water, there is less disruption to your stroke and rhythm.

Strong swimmers also don't turn their heads that much to breathe. Rather, they rotate their torso and the head stays in line with the upper body. Only about half the face emerges from the water and hardly any head turning is required to do this. Check out the goggles of elite swimmers as they breathe. Often, only one lens emerges from the water.

Efficient breathing in front crawl is a hard skill to master, so don't expect immediate results. Find easy ways to practise. For example, in the shallow end of a swimming pool, while standing on the bottom, lean forwards, lower your face into the water and gently breath out. Then, still in the shallow end and standing, rotate your shoulders and head to one side. Try to keep one eye under the water. Imagine a line through the centre of your face running from your chin to your forehead. When you breathe, align that line with the water level. Try to breathe in by opening the half of your mouth that's above the water. This is the position you should aim for while swimming.

Next, try floating face down in the water, holding the wall with one hand and with the other hand by your side. You can kick your legs gently to keep them near the surface. Now try to breathe again by putting your head in the same position. Finally, try to achieve the same thing while swimming.

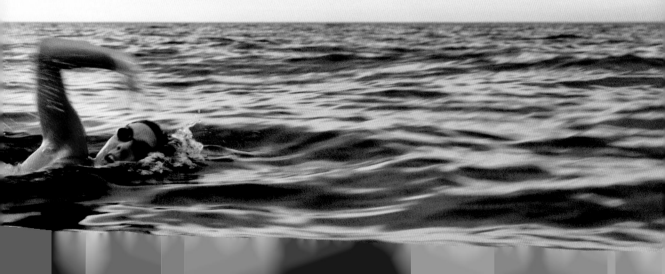

Single-sided or bilateral breathing?

You can either breathe constantly on the same side or you can switch between left and right side breathing. The latter is known as bilateral breathing. The most usual pattern with bilateral breathing is to breathe every three strokes, but other patterns are possible. A lot of energy is spent on discussing the pros and cons of each. The bottom line is that while being able to breathe on both sides clearly gives you more options, it's not a disaster if you only ever breathe to one side. I know plenty of brilliant swimmers who only breathe to one side and nothing bad has happened to them because of it, so don't lose sleep over it if you can only breathe one way.

That said, it's worth practising breathing both sides, because it can help remove asymmetries from your stroke and it may be useful when swimming outside. For example, if the sun is low on the horizon you might want to look away from it, or you may be swimming parallel to the shore and want to keep an eye on it. In a race situation, it will help you watch your competitors.

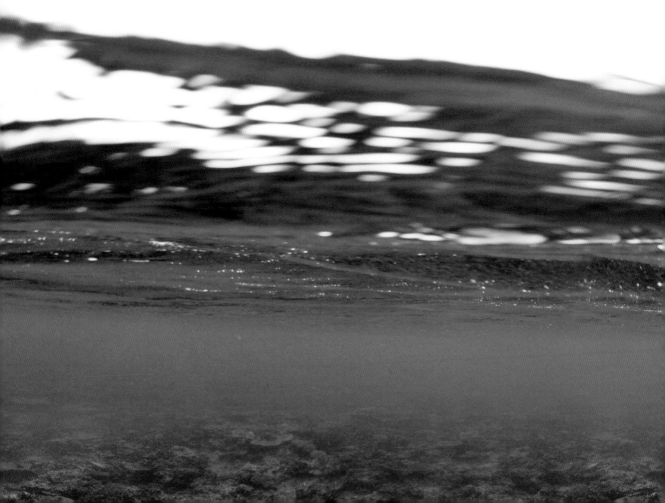

Legs

Legs cause beginner swimmers lots of problems. Not only do they often tend to sink, but they also frequently move in other undesirable ways, such as excessive bending at the knee and swinging sideways. Many people have inflexible ankles, meaning their feet stay at a right angle to their legs.

As discussed earlier, sinking legs are usually a symptom of some other issue with the stroke rather than a problem of the legs themselves. Similarly, the cause of legs swinging side to side or separating too widely is found elsewhere. For example, your legs may swing sideways to counterbalance an incorrect arm movement. Then, however much you try to point your toes, it's not going to happen unless you have sufficient flexibility in the first place. Nobody said this was going to be easy.

The action you carry out with your legs while swimming is generally referred to as kicking, but it's not the same action as kicking a football. Instead, the legs move alternately, in a short swinging motion starting from the hips. The knee bends very little. The feet are stretched with the toes pointing away from the direction of travel.

Sprint swimmers can generate significant propulsion with their legs, but only for short distances. Distance swimmers tend to use them more for balance. Kicking hard consumes a lot of energy. Unless you have a very effective kick, most of that energy will be wasted. It can even be counter-productive.

The best approach for beginner and intermediate swimmers is therefore often to minimise the potential problems caused by legs rather than trying to increase propulsion. Focus on keeping them straight but relaxed. If they are sinking or swinging from side to side, look for the cause elsewhere rather than trying to fix it by kicking harder.

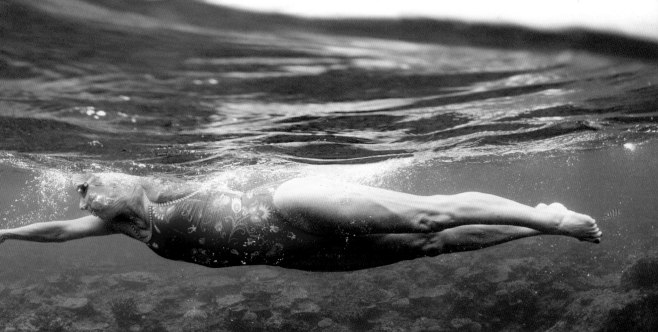

Pull buoys, kickboards and swim fins

PULL BUOYS
In training, you may see swimmers using a special float between their legs, known as a pull buoy. These do a great job of disguising some of the problems swimmers have with legs. They lift them higher in the water and force you to keep them closer together. They can be useful in helping you get a sense of what good body and leg position feels like, or allowing you to focus on correct breathing or arm movements. However, swimming is a full-body activity and needs to be practised as such, so use the pull buoy sparingly and don't use it as a speed booster in training.

KICKBOARDS
Another float you see swimmers use is a large, flat one called a kickboard. This is usually held out in front with both hands, sometimes with the arms resting on the float, and allows you to practise kicking without using your arms. However, as the float stops you rotating, it disconnects your body movements from your leg movements and changes your body position in the water, so I see this more as a fitness exercise than one to improve your leg kick.

SWIM FINS
Swim fins – small flippers used by swimmers – can be useful in helping improve ankle flexibility, so might be worth experimenting with for that. They can also help with some swimming drills where you need a little extra propulsion.

Kick timing and connection

The two most common timings in front crawl kicking are known as two-beat and six-beat. In two-beat kicking, you get one kick with each arm stroke (so two kicks for the complete arm cycle) and in six-beat kicking, you get three kicks for each arm stroke. You will probably find that you have already adopted one of these two patterns automatically. Try to work out which one you do by paying attention next time you swim. Sprinters usually use a six-beat kick. Long-distance swimmers may use either a two-beat kick or a light six-beat kick.

Whichever kicking pattern you use, it will be more effective if it is connected and co-ordinated with the rest of your body. This may or may not happen naturally. I needed a coach and a lot of practice to get this right. Some people have never thought about it and it works fine.

In a two-beat kick, the right leg 'kicks' (think of it more of a toe flick, the end result of a downward movement initiated at your hips) at the same time as three other movements:

1. Your body rotating from its right side to its left.
2. Your left hand and arm entering the water and sliding forwards.
3. Your right hand and arm pressing back against the water as they pass under your chest.

You then mirror this for the left foot.

In a six-beat kick, two kicks are stronger than the others and these coincide with the timing of the single-beat kick. In between, you have two smaller, lighter kicks, one with each foot.

Arms

I've deliberately left arms until last as people often focus on them first, since they are the main providers of propulsion in front crawl. However, if you don't have a streamlined body position, a lot of the effort you put in through your arms will be wasted. Before bringing in your arms spend time feeling how changes in your head position affect your legs and how to use your legs effectively.

I would then spend some time on YouTube browsing videos of elite swimmers, or watch Swim Smooth's animations. These will help you visualise what you should be doing. However, bear in mind that whole books have been written on this topic.

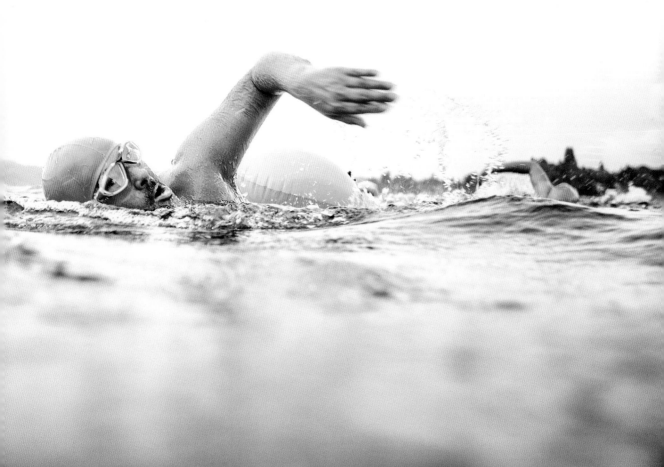

Here are a few pointers to get you started:

1. To move forwards, you need to press the water backwards – not downwards or sideways.
2. You achieve this by bending the elbow at the front of the stroke so that your palm is facing backwards, then press through in a straight line until it's roughly level with your hips.
3. Remember that at the same time your hand is pressing back, your foot on the same side is kicking and you are rotating on to your other side.
4. Once the hand has reached your hips, pull it straight out of the water and swing it forwards. This is called the recovery phase. Your hand and arm should be relaxed, with your hand lower than your elbow.
5. Your hand re-enters the water a short distance in front of your head and in line with your shoulder.
6. Your fingertips enter first, then the rest of your arm follows through. As your arm straightens in front of your head, keep your fingertips lower than your wrist and your wrist lower than your elbow.
7. Your arms move alternately but they are not opposites. Start the stroke of your right arm roughly as your left arm enters the water, and vice versa, so that your arms spend more time in front of your head than behind.

Other key factors with front crawl include stroke rate and rhythm. In simple terms, your speed through the water is determined by how far you move with each stroke (which in turn is a factor of power versus drag or resistance) and how quickly you take your strokes. There is a lot of variation between swimmers for these factors. Experiment with your stroke rates and time yourself with a stopwatch to see what happens to your speed.

Rhythm is related to stroke rate, but, for me, it also describes the feeling when everything about my stroke is working as it should be and it all feels co-ordinated. It's a great feeling and something to strive for while swimming.

As you can see, there's a lot more to swimming technique than you might at first think. The above is merely a brief look at this fascinating topic, and only for one of the strokes. I hope you're inspired to explore it further. In your research, you will come across a number of different teaching methodologies and philosophies. You may also find conflicting advice and a range of opinions, and you will have to use your own judgement to decide which works best for you.

Two of the better-known approaches have been developed by the late Terry Laughlin at Total Immersion, and Paul Newsome and Adam Young with Swim Smooth. Both are worth looking at.

PHYSICAL FITNESS AND YOUR SWIM-SPECIFIC FITNESS

To swim well and maintain your pace, you need a special type of fitness that you can only get by swimming.

You can be fit and strong, yet still swim slowly and get exhausted quickly if you have poor swimming technique, which is why learning and refining good stroke mechanics is so important. If you want to become a better swimmer, prioritise technique over fitness every time. Developing good swimming technique will always help you swim faster and further. Improving your fitness will also help you swim faster and further, but the gains are only temporary. Lose your fitness and your speed will decrease. Fitness declines much faster than the muscle memory for good swimming technique.

That said, having a good fitness base will help your swimming, so it pays to work on it. Swimmers also recognise something we refer to as 'swimming fitness', which you only get from spending time in the water. Through lockdown, when pools where closed and it was too cold for training in the open water, I stayed fit through running and trying to replicate swimming-specific movements on land using stretch cords. When I got back to the water, I was fit and I'd maintained strength in my arms and shoulders, yet I was significantly slower because I'd lost swim-specific fitness.

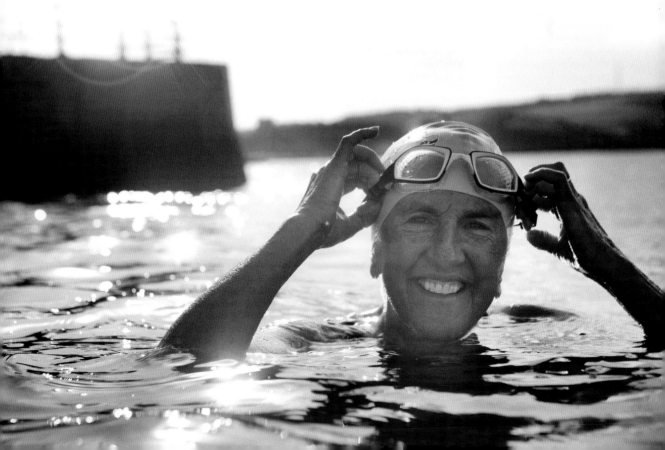

General Health

At first, simply working on your swimming technique and spending time in the water will improve both your general and swim-specific fitness. You don't need to do anything special. However, if this is all you do, you will hit a plateau at which you don't make more progress. At this point, you may want to look at what else you can do. There are several strands to pursue here and, again, this book is only an introduction.

The first step is to do your best to put in place good foundations by eating well and getting sufficient sleep. This is easier said than done, I know, but most of us are aware of how to eat properly and the importance of sleep. You don't need to be extreme with this, but stay alert to what you eat and the quality of your sleep. Although outdoor swimmers are fond of cake, becoming a swimmer and doing some training is not a licence to eat whatever you fancy. Indulge in some post-swim cake by all means, but make sure the rest of your diet includes plenty of fresh food.

A quick note about weight, body shape and swimming is in order here. Carrying a little extra weight has one very clear advantage in outdoor swimming: it can help keep you warmer in cool water for longer. And, unlike, say, running or cycling, extra weight has only a limited impact on your swimming speed. This makes outdoor swimming a very welcoming sport for a wide range of body types. People training for long-distance swims in cool water often try to put on weight to reduce the risk of hypothermia.

The key point is that you don't need to get in shape, lose weight or gain weight before you start outdoor swimming. The activity and exercise will be good for you, regardless of your body type.

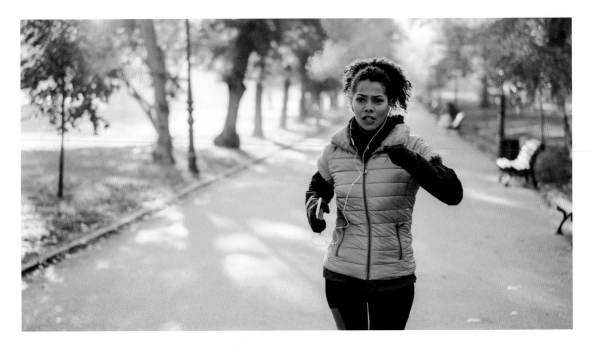

Land Training

Step two in your swimming fitness journey also has nothing to do with the water. Elite swimmers do a substantial amount of training on land, such as shifting weights in a gym or doing circuits. They will have a training programme designed to target specific muscle groups to help them swim faster and reduce injury risk.

For recreational swimmers, you don't need a dedicated gym programme, but anything that improves and sustains mobility and core strength will be a big help for your swimming. Pilates and yoga are both popular. Dancing would be good. Running and cycling can help with your cardiovascular fitness. Hitting the gym is also fine, but make sure you include core and mobility exercises. If you intend to do a serious amount of swimming, add some specific exercises to reduce the risk of shoulder injury.

In the Water

The third part of swimming fitness is what you do in the water. When you first start, simply swimming up and down the pool or doing circuits in a lake will improve your fitness. You'll learn how to relax and swim within your comfort zone. You should quite easily be able to increase the distance you swim. At some point, however, you may decide you want to do some swim training, rather than just swimming. Remember, there is no compulsion to do this. Outdoor swimming can be enjoyed equally well whether you're fast or slow, fit or unfit.

> **Three reasons to try swim training:**
>
> **1.** Training is fun, even when it's hard work.
> **2.** Training helps you swim faster, which is satisfying.
> **3.** Training builds your strength and fitness more quickly than just swimming.

If you decide you want to try swim training, then there are a number of ways to access it. One is through a masters swimming club. Masters in this context means any swimmer over the age of 25, although most masters clubs will be open to anyone over the age of 18. If you swam with a club as a child, then you'll be familiar with the type of training you do in a club. The advantages of swimming with a club are that it is social and there is often a coach designing the sessions. The disadvantage is that the training might not match your needs (it's often designed around sprint training for pool races, for example). Also, the standard of swimming is often high and you may need to develop your swimming skills elsewhere before you can keep up.

Another option is to look for swim fit classes or similar. These are generally aimed at adult learners and improvers rather than people who swam with clubs as children. These may offer more stroke improvement tuition than a masters club, too.

Both masters clubs and swim fit groups tend to do the bulk of their training in a pool, although you may be lucky to find a group that trains outdoors.

The third option is to join a triathlon group or club. You'll need to check if that's cost-effective if you're only going to swim, but often the bulk of the costs to the club are in swimming provision, so this could be a good option. Triathlon groups are used to helping non-swimming adults take to the water and may have sessions both in pools and in open water.

Finally, you can design your own training routines and do them in a public session. It's easy to find examples of training sessions and plans on the internet, so I haven't included any here, but note that generic plans won't have been made specifically for you, so make sure you adapt and modify them to suit your circumstances.

Designing Your Own Training Plans and Sessions

Training is normally designed around a goal – typically an event at some date in the not-too-distant future – as this helps you create a structure or a training plan. A training plan is a series of swimming sessions that are designed to maximise your performance in your goal event.

You can also train for general fitness, without a specific goal in mind. In this case, there will be less of a structure between sessions, although you may still want to try to build in progression by, for example, increasing the distance you swim in a session over a number of weeks. You might find, as I do, that you spend part of the year training for general fitness. You then fix on an event or swim challenge that you'd like to do, which brings focus to your training and allows you to create a plan.

It also depends on what motivates you. Some people enjoy the variety and flexibility of the general fitness approach. Other people like the incentive of a challenge to work towards.

There is no right or wrong here and there are advantages and disadvantages to both. For example, the challenge approach might inspire a big increase in training and improvement in fitness, but maybe then leave you directionless and demotivated when it's done.

That said, it is easier to design a training plan when you have an end goal in mind. For example, if you decide you want to complete a half-marathon 5km (3.1-mile) swim in four months, you might create a training plan that includes a long continuous swim each week, perhaps starting with 1km (0.6 miles) and building up to 4 or 5km (2.5–3.1 miles) over 16 weeks. You might also build in some training sessions that help you practise swimming at your target pace and help you increase the distance you can maintain that pace for.

As an outdoor swimmer, most events you do will be endurance challenges. High-volume, low-intensity swimming is the best way to build your endurance, so make this part of your training. I always like to add in a few sprints, too, and I practise all four competitive swimming strokes (butterfly, backstroke, breaststroke and front crawl) for variety and the overall fitness benefits.

You should always concentrate on swimming with good technique, but it can also be useful to incorporate specific exercises (coaches usually refer to them as 'drills') into your training to help improve any weaknesses. But make sure you know what purpose any drills you do serve.

Every time you swim, regardless of whether or not you have a long-term training plan or if you're swimming for pleasure and general fitness, it's worth spending a few minutes thinking through what you will do when you hit the water. It might help to write this down.

How to create your own training session plan

Designing your own training sessions and plans is easy, and you can make them specific to your goals. Here's how to go about it. If I'm training in a pool, I find it best to write or print out a session plan, put it in a waterproof see-through plastic bag, and place it at the end of the lane for reference while swimming.

PRE SWIM

Spend 5–10 minutes loosening up on land before you get in the water. This is especially useful if you've just got out of bed or you've spent the day hunched over a computer. Gentle shoulder rolls, arm swings, leg swings and trunk rotations are all you need. It makes a difference to how you feel in the water.

WARM UP

Most swim training sessions start with a warm-up. I like to use this time as a mental warm-up as much as a physical one. Spend about 5–10 minutes swimming at a gentle pace. Relax and enjoy the sensation of being in the water. Think through any key swimming technique points you're working on and try to incorporate those as you swim. When swimming outside, use this time to adjust to the water temperature. If you're wearing a wetsuit, make sure it's fitted properly and is not rubbing your neck or anywhere else.

MAIN SECTION

This is where you see the most variety. The main section of your training could consist of one big training set or a series of small sets. Some coaches set aside time at the beginning for technique exercises. I have a personal preference for keeping things simple and repetitive. For example, in a pool session, I might do 16 lots of 100m (110 yards) with a few seconds' rest between each one, or 6 lots of 400m (440 yards) with 30 seconds' rest after each one. Other people don't enjoy swimming like this and prefer to mix things up more. In practice, your session will probably end up as a compromise between the following factors:

- What's best for your swimming goals.
- What you want to do and enjoy.
- What the people you are swimming with want to do.
- What is practical to do in a public session, if you're swimming in a pool.

COOL DOWN

This is the bit where you get to relax and unwind after all the hard work. If you like, flip on to your back and watch the clouds. Let your heart rate come down and your breathing get back to normal.

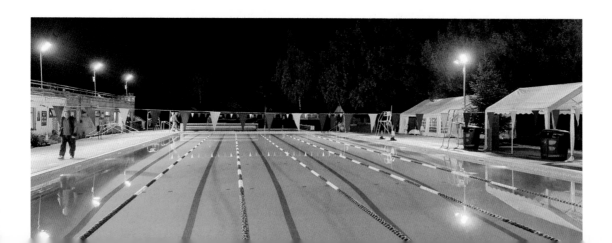

Putting Sessions into a Plan

For general fitness and variety, you might want to mix your sessions up so that one day you focus on endurance in your main set, another day you work on sustainable speed and perhaps do sprints on a third. A rough rule of thumb among swimmers is that you can maintain your fitness with one to two sessions per week, but you need three or more if you want to make improvements. However, this will obviously depend on your current fitness and abilities. If you are starting from zero, then you will make improvements with one session a week. An elite swimmer would lose fitness if they only did three sessions per week. For recreational swimmers, three or four shorter sessions per week will be more effective than one long one.

When designing a plan for a specific challenge, work back from the date of the event to where you are now. This might be 12 weeks for a 1-mile (1.6km) swim or two years for swimming the English Channel. Then plot out a plan that incrementally advances your swim fitness towards that goal. Every three or four weeks, allow for a few easy sessions and extra rest, as recovery is important. About a week to 10 days before your challenge, scale back the training (but don't stop) so that you're fresh on the day.

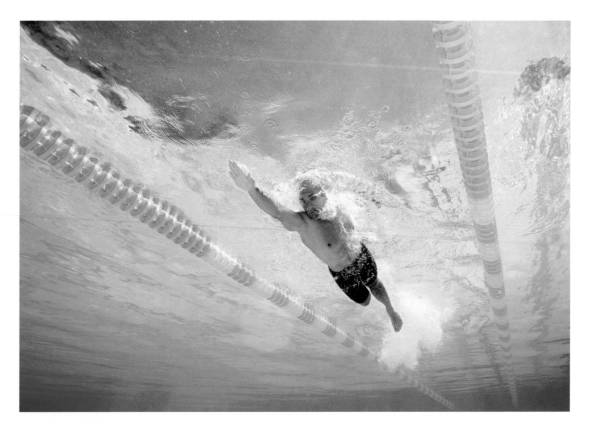

MY STORY

Building a life around swimming

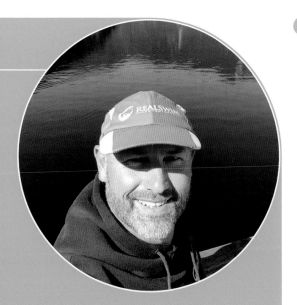

On a trip to London I ran into some chaps preparing for an English Channel relay who needed some help. I ended up joining the team and attribute much of my love of outdoor swimming to that open water event. This swim challenge was not about laps, times and perfection. Instead, it was about temperature, nature, the environment and enjoyment. A switch was triggered. This is what I wanted to do. I loved swimming in open water and I loved helping those who didn't know of it and hadn't experienced it to find this joy.

In February 2011, I was visiting my native New Zealand when we experienced our worst modern-day earthquake in my home city of Christchurch. I was up in the hills at the time, having just been out surfing. I didn't know until much later that I suffered from PTSD for some time after. But I did realise our city needed help. I couldn't rebuild houses, but I knew outdoor swimming was great for taking our minds off stress, healing, connecting with nature and as a way to make friends. I therefore set about finding ways to introduce as many people to outdoor swimming as possible.

Our relationship with water runs deep. It allows us to experience low gravity without going to the moon. It has mental healing powers science still doesn't fully understand. It allows us to connect deeply with the environment. It can be fun, scary or relaxing. It can help clear our thoughts; to refresh and begin anew while at the same time viewing the world from a different perspective. I get joy out of doing open water swimming. I get joy out of helping others learn to enjoy the experience. I get joy out of helping others connect with nature via the water.

DAN ABEL

COPING WITH CONDITIONS

Pools are adapted for human comfort and safety. When you step outside, it's you that has to adapt to whatever nature sends your way.

The third pillar of training for outdoor swimming is learning to cope with conditions. An indoor pool is nearly always the same warm temperature. The water is calm. There's no wind blowing waves in your face. You're unlikely to be dazzled by the sun. You won't touch a leaf and panic that it's a shark or a jellyfish. That all changes when you get outside. Learning to cope with the differences is primarily a question of experience. The more swimming outside you do, and the more different conditions you swim in, the better you'll be able to cope. Remember, coping is just the first phase. You may well come to love getting cold and playing in the waves. But let's have a look at how you might speed up the learning process.

Cold

We've looked at the cold already, in Chapter 6. To recap, there are essentially two components to coping with cold water: (1) your initial response, which lasts a couple of minutes; and (2) your longer-term ability to withstand the cold, for anything from 10 minutes to multiple hours. These two components are not strongly correlated.

Your initial response to cold water is extremely adaptable. Most people can significantly reduce the impact of cold water shock after a few immersions, as discussed earlier. As far as I've observed, anyone, regardless of body size and shape, can learn to tolerate (even enjoy) immersion in cold water for a short period of time.

On the other hand, you see a lot more diversity in people's ability to stay warm for longer periods, not just in the extremes of winter, but also in the still-cool coastal and inland waters of summer. While you can acclimatise and improve your tolerance of cold water to an extent, and learn to be more comfortable when you are cold, body size and shape are bigger factors – marathon swimmers try to put on weight for a reason.

Personally, I've no time for tough talking around cold water tolerance. The potential consequences of hypothermia are too serious. You can't push through hypothermia. Mental toughness will get you into difficulties.

Without invasive tools (e.g. a thermometer up your rectum) it's hard to get an accurate measure of your core temperature when swimming. As one of the effects of acclimatisation is that you become more comfortable with a depressed core body temperature, how you feel is not a good guide.

Keep a record of water temperatures and swimming times, and note how long it takes you to recover after your swim. Your recovery time is a useful (but not infallible) guide to how cold you got. If you were completely fine 15 minutes after a swim and didn't shiver, you could swim for longer at that temperature (but you don't have to). If you were a shivering wreck for 20–30 minutes, then you've overdone it. Through keeping a record, you will learn what you can do and monitor any changes.

Try not to pay too much heed to what other people do and avoid involvement in any macho boasting about staying in X temperature water for Y minutes. Always give yourself a wide margin for error as your temperature tolerance can change depending on a range of internal and external factors.

A wetsuit gives you additional protection from the cold and you can put on additional layers and accessories as you need. However, before adding layers and accessories, I would do a few swims. You should find that the discomfort you may initially experience in your hands and feet disappears quickly, and you might not need the extra kit.

Waves and Rough Water

Waves are fascinating and can be fun to swim in. They can also be tiresome and, in extreme cases, dangerous. They are mostly associated with sea, but you find waves on lakes and rivers, too.

Mostly, waves are generated by wind blowing across the water surface. The size of the waves is determined by multiple factors, including the wind speed, the amount of time it blows for and the surface area of water the wind blows over. A gentle wind produces ripples that remain local and vanish if the wind drops. Stronger winds produce larger waves that can travel thousands of miles from where they were generated. Once waves move away from the area they were generated, we refer to them as swell.

When waves approach land, interesting things start to happen. On gently sloping beaches, they turn into surf. If they hit cliffs, they reflect back and then interfere with fresh oncoming waves. Waves arriving from across

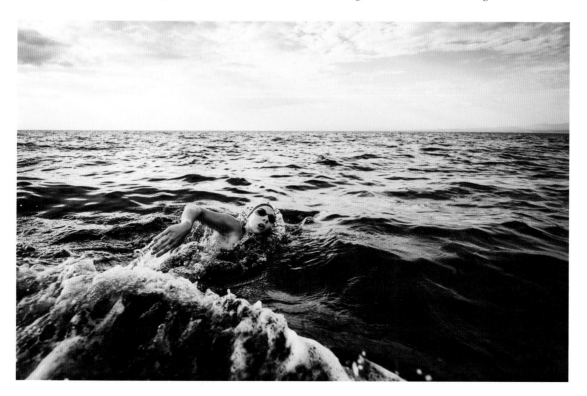

the ocean are also affected by local conditions. This is easily seen on surfing beaches where an offshore wind helps stack the waves into neat breakers that surfers love. When the wind is blowing in from the sea, chasing the waves, they become messy and choppy.

The best way to become more confident about swimming in waves is to do it often. Start by playing in waves on a lifeguarded beach (swim in the area set aside for swimmers to ensure you don't collide with a surfer). To swim out to sea through the waves, try diving underneath the crests. Have a go at bodysurfing. Find the point where the wave crests are about to topple, wait for a suitable wave and start swimming towards shore just in front of it. If you get the timing right, the wave will pick you up and shoot you down the front face. Lift your head to see where you're going, leave one arm stretched out in front with your hand open, skimming across the water. Use the other arm to steer and provide extra propulsion if needed.

Some care is needed. Make sure you swim on a beach that doesn't have underwater obstacles such as reefs you might crash into. The waves need to be 50cm (20in) tall or so to have enough power to surf on, but if they get too big things get scary. A large wave breaking over your head will tumble you around and hold you under. If this happens, try to stay calm. Once the energy of the wave has dissipated, you will get back to the surface.

Swimming, as opposed to playing, is a different proposition, but the more you play in the waves, the easier you will find swimming in them. Once you're past the breakers, swimming into waves is easy enough but you may need to adjust the timing of your stroke to match the ups and downs. Lift your head at the top of the wave to see where you're going. It will feel like your progress is slow when swimming into the waves, but push on. It may help if you swim harder going up the wave and then relax on the way back down.

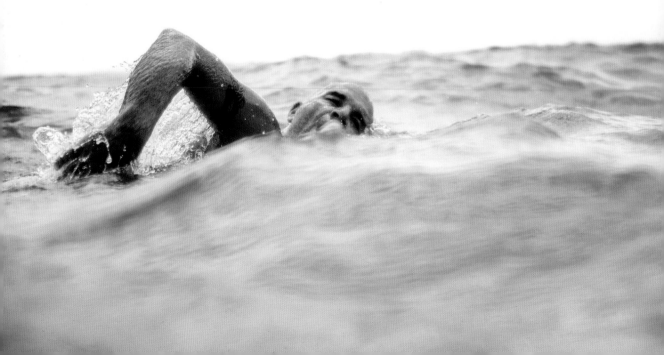

Going in the same direction as the waves is more fun as you get a free ride when a wave picks you up and carries you forwards, although the sensation takes some getting used to. It's worth practising and paying attention as you can sometimes increase the boost by changing your effort levels. Swim harder when the wave is carrying you. Once the wave has passed, you'll feel a lull. Relax rather than fighting it and wait for the next wave to roll along and give you a ride.

When swimming sideways in waves, you may want to change the side you breathe so you can see the waves coming, or else turn away from the waves to avoid getting smacked in the face. You'll have to see what works best in the circumstances. Try to get a feel for the timing of the waves. You may find adjusting the rhythm of your stroke to the pattern of the waves makes swimming easier.

In general, I find it more comfortable to relax and stay calm when swimming in waves, especially as they become less predictable. Trying to fight your way through quickly becomes exhausting. However, if you are fit and have practised it, increasing your stroke rate and developing a strong rhythm can be a good way to punch through.

Chop

We use the term 'chop' or 'choppy' to describe a water surface that's roughed up with lots of small waves that don't have any particular sense of direction. Chop is usually generated by local wind conditions, whereas waves have travelled in from elsewhere. You can have chop on top of waves.

Chop is often a feature on rivers and lakes, too, and can be disruptive to your swimming as it feels random. A combination of strong rhythm in your stroke and a calm mindset will help you get through it. Be prepared for the occasional wave smacking you in the face when sighting or trying to breathe. If it happens, try to keep your rhythm, take another stroke and try again.

Currents

We've already looked at the risks with currents, but just because they present a potential hazard doesn't mean you can't swim in them. Swooshing along with a current is one of the joys of outdoor swimming. In events, you can sometimes use currents to your advantage. For example, in rivers, the current tends to be strongest towards the middle and on the outside of bends. This knowledge can help you both swimming up or downstream. Likewise, if you're swimming along the coast and there is a current, this tends to be stronger further away from the coast.

Observe how currents swirl and even reverse as they encounter obstacles and use that to your advantage, too. Watch how the water piles up in front of a bridge pillar in a river on the upstream side and notice the patch of calm water on the downstream side. If the currents are strong, it's best to stay away from obstacles as you can get pinned against them or pushed underneath them.

In the sea and estuaries, the currents change with the tides. Take a look at local tide tables before swimming to make sure you get your timing right.

OPEN WATER SKILLS

Mastering a few simple skills will make your outdoor swimming more efficient and enjoyable. If you want to race, they will make you faster.

Open water skills – such as sighting, drafting and turns – don't just happen. You need to work on them to do them well. If you spend your winter swimming in a pool and never practise open water skills, they go rusty between seasons. I find that if I haven't practised sighting for a while, my neck and back get tired quickly when I first return to open water. You don't need a lot of practice to keep the skills fresh, but here are a couple of things you can do.

Sighting and Swimming Straight

In a swimming pool, you usually have a black line or tiles to follow, and lane ropes to keep you on the straight and narrow. Outdoors, you often can't see the bottom and there are no ropes or walls. If you put your head down and swim front crawl you will most likely veer off course within a few strokes. Try it out one day. It will be an interesting experiment and it's useful to know if you have a tendency to drift left or right. To counter this, when swimming front crawl outdoors, you need to look up from time to time to see where you're going. Swimmers refer to this as 'sighting'.

Breaststroke swimmers should have no trouble swimming straight as they can look where they are going on every stroke, but front crawl swimmers need to incorporate sighting into their stroke. There are different ways to do this, so experiment and see what is most comfortable and efficient for you. My preference is to lift my head to look forwards just before I breathe.

This means that if you're about to breathe to your left, lift your head as your right arm is in the air and swinging forwards. At the same time, you can press down slightly with your left hand as it starts the stroke, to help with raising your head. After a brief glance, drop your head back into its neutral face down position at the same time as your right hand is entering the water, then take your breath on the left normally. Mirror the above if you're breathing to the right.

Only lift your head as high as you need to. In flat water, you can get away with your eyes clearing the water. If it's choppy, you may need to lift a little higher. The higher you lift your head, the more you disrupt the rhythm of your stroke and put strain on your neck and lower back.

Do not pause the sighting movement if you don't see what you expect or hope to see. Instead, repeat it on the next stroke and look in a slightly different direction. It's better not to panic and to keep the rhythm of your stroke going if you can.

If you still haven't seen what you need to see after three or four attempts, try holding your head up while you take a few strokes, as if you were swimming water polo. If this doesn't work, then you may have to switch to breaststroke for a few strokes or even stop to look around – but this doesn't happen very often.

How often you sight depends on the conditions, how straight you swim, how close you are to other swimmers and how important it is that you hold your line. Sighting slows you down, but so does swimming off course and adding to the total distance. You need to find a balance that works for you in the situation you're in. Coming up to a turn in a race, I might sight every other stroke to make sure I get the best line through the turn. If the next marker is several hundred metres/yards away, I might swim 20 strokes without looking up.

With practice, you should be able to incorporate sighting smoothly into your stroke so that it becomes part of your rhythm and not a break in it. Since lifting your head to sight causes your legs to sink, experiment with doing one or two harder kicks to maintain your body position.

Sighting practice in the pool

There is no need to sight when swimming in a pool as most have black lines on the bottom you can follow. You may have noticed that these black lines usually end in a 'T'. This tells you the wall is approaching and you need to turn. You don't need to look forwards at all.

To practise sighting while in the pool, lift your head once a length and look forwards. It might help to have something at the end of the pool, such as your water bottle, to look for and focus on. Also scan left to right, as if you're looking for a marker buoy. You don't need to do this all the time, but maybe designate a portion of your swim when you will practise sighting.

As well as trying to spot whatever you're trying to see, work on keeping the action as smooth as possible. Make it an integrated, flowing part of your stroke so you don't lose any momentum. How low can you lift your eyes and still see what you need to? Can you get just your eyes out of the water and leave your nose and mouth under the water? Practise sighting when you're breathing both to the left and the right. Is one side easier for you than the other?

Drafting

Drafting is a technique that is used in open water racing to save energy or swim faster. This is covered in more detail in the next chapter, but in essence it involves swimming in the slipstream of another swimmer, either behind their feet or next to their hip. It is harder to practise in a pool than outdoors as you need to find someone who is willing to have you swim closely behind. Don't practise drafting strangers in the pool.

In organised training sessions, the usual etiquette is to leave 5 or 10 seconds and swimmers can get annoyed if you don't observe this. With a five-second gap, you will still get some drafting benefit, but it's not the same as swimming right behind someone's feet. The best way to practise in the pool then is to swim with a friend and make sure you have their permission to swim right behind them. Pay attention at the turns to ensure you don't have a painful collision. If you want to practise drafting next to someone's hip in a pool, you need a lane to yourself or to do it as part of an organised open water skills session.

In open water, in a non-competitive situation, drafting strangers is also impolite, although people do it. It's much better to rope in a few friends and take it in turns leading and drafting in different positions. When drafting next to someone's hip, you may need to change your stroke rate to match theirs to avoid clashing arms. Try to get a feeling of how the draft effect changes depending on where you swim.

When it's your turn to take the lead, swim as normal. You don't need to make any concessions to people drafting in your wake. It may feel like people on your feet are slowing you down, as if you're dragging them, but that's not the case. In fact, the lead swimmer also benefits and swims faster for the same effort when someone is drafting behind them.

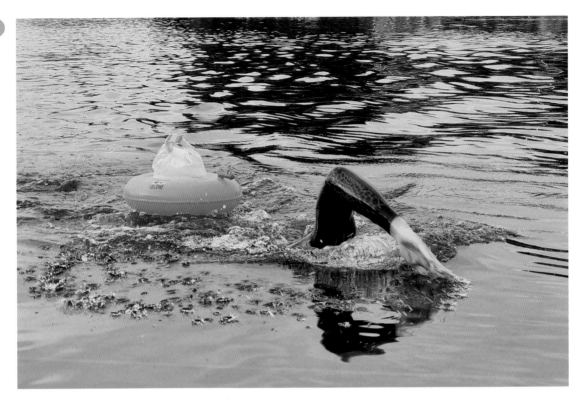

Open Water Turns

You only need to worry about open water turns – the art of changing swimming direction without losing speed – if you are planning to race. See the section in the next chapter on racing for details on how to execute a slick turn in open water, where you have no wall to bounce off. The most obvious place to practise open water turns is a venue marked out with buoys, as that's the closest you will find to a racing scenario.

In the pool, especially if you're swimming in a narrow single lane, it's awkward as you have to turn 180 degrees, which is more than you will usually encounter in a race. Still, it's good to get used to the idea of turning without touching or pushing off the wall. Work on getting back into your normal swimming position as quickly as possible after the turn to regain any lost momentum.

Wearing a Wetsuit

Making the most of the advantages offered by a wetsuit takes a little experience, so it is worth practising. Firstly, this means putting it on properly. Once in the water, notice how the wetsuit changes your body position. Because of the (slight) restriction to your shoulder mobility, experiment with a slightly wider arm recovery than you might use in the pool. Do you need to kick so hard when wearing a wetsuit? Try it and see. You may find you can almost stop kicking and save yourself lots of energy.

If you've got an event or challenge coming up at which you'll be wearing a wetsuit, swim in it first to get used to the differences, even if that means taking it to the pool. Remember, though, that indoor pool temperatures are maintained at at least 26°C (78.8°F) and you will overheat in a wetsuit if you keep it on for too long. Test it and then remove it to continue your swim, and rinse it well in fresh water afterwards.

MENTAL PREPARATION

Whatever your swim challenge, having your mind in the right place could make a big difference to your success and enjoyment of it.

As well as preparing physically for an open water swim, preparing your mind can make a big difference to how you feel and perform at your event. This is a huge and fascinating topic that you may want to research further. To get you started, here are some of the things I incorporate into my training.

Visualisation

When you swim, you have to co-ordinate lots of different parts of your body. Unlike moving on land, you have nothing to fix yourself against. Trying to think about all of this while in the water can cause confusion and co-ordination failures. If I'm trying to make an improvement I will therefore try to imagine

and feel it in slow motion while I'm on land. I also visualise how I'm going to approach an open water swim. I imagine myself feeling confident and strong in the water. Numerous studies have demonstrated the positive power of visualisation. It's not a substitute for getting in the water and swimming, but it's a useful complement.

Visualisation is also a useful technique to practise in the run-up to a big event or challenge. Imagine yourself at the event, getting changed, entering the water, swimming and finishing. Feel yourself carving through the water, perhaps overtaking your rivals in a sprint finish. If you do this well, you can actually feel your heart rate increase and the adrenaline pumping.

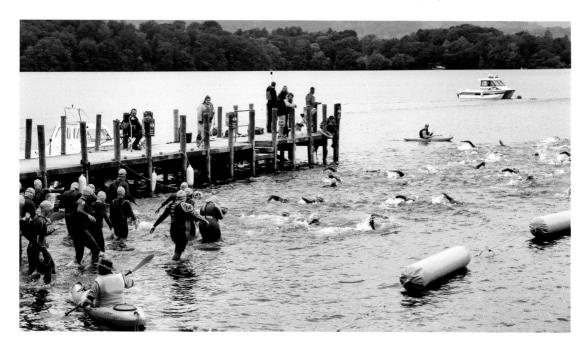

Mantras

A mantra is a word or phrase you repeat to yourself. In a sporting context, it's something to help you stay focused. For example, I use the single word 'relax' in both training and in an event, to remind myself to relax my arms on the recovery part of the stroke. I have a habit of holding my breath when I put my face in the water, rather than letting it out gently. I sometimes therefore repeat: 'Relax. Breathe.' This reminds me to relax and breathe out. Alternatively, try a confidence-boosting mantra such as 'You've got this' to help you through a tough training session or section of a race.

Visual Reminders of What You've Done

In the days and moments leading up to a big swim, it's normal to start worrying about the training you haven't done, the sessions you missed because of work deadlines, the days you didn't have the energy. It's more beneficial to remind yourself of what you have done, yet for some reason the few training sessions we've missed seem to weigh more heavily on our minds than the many we've completed. The first step is to keep a record. You can do this on a wall chart, in a spreadsheet or on an app – whichever works for you. Then, when you're feeling nervous, look at the records so you can see what you've done. Obviously, you have to have done the training in the first place, but having a chart to fill in can help with the motivation for that, too.

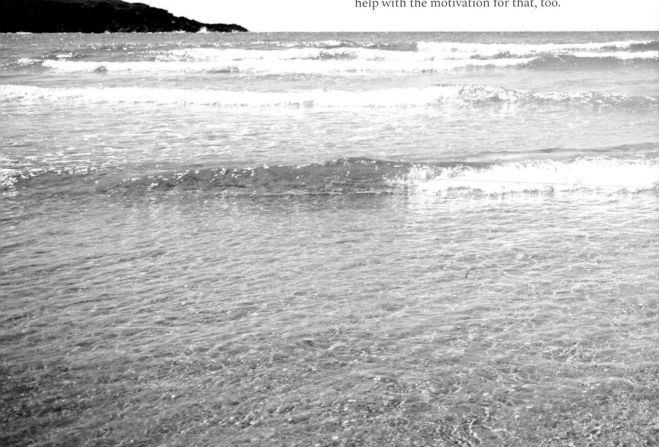

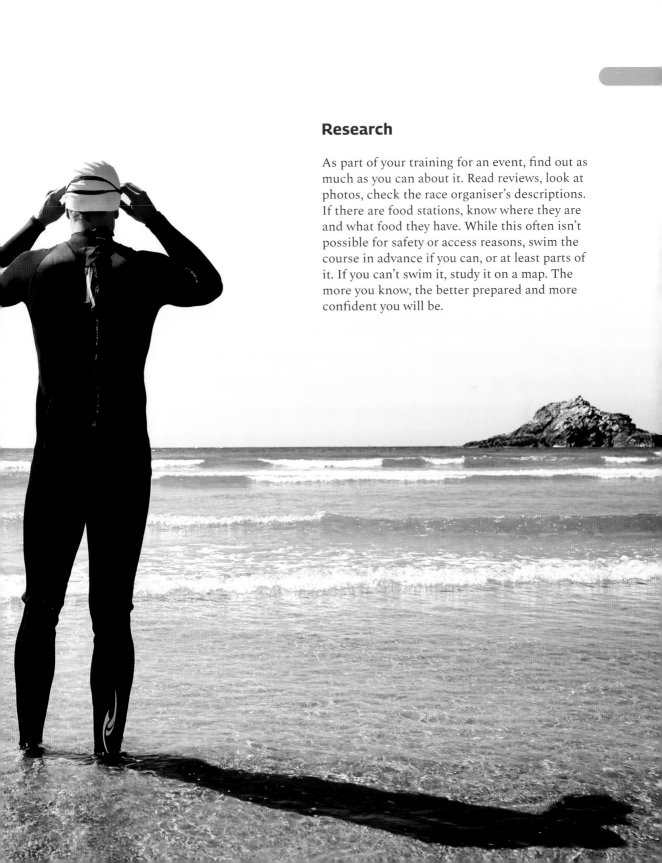

Research

As part of your training for an event, find out as much as you can about it. Read reviews, look at photos, check the race organiser's descriptions. If there are food stations, know where they are and what food they have. While this often isn't possible for safety or access reasons, swim the course in advance if you can, or at least parts of it. If you can't swim it, study it on a map. The more you know, the better prepared and more confident you will be.

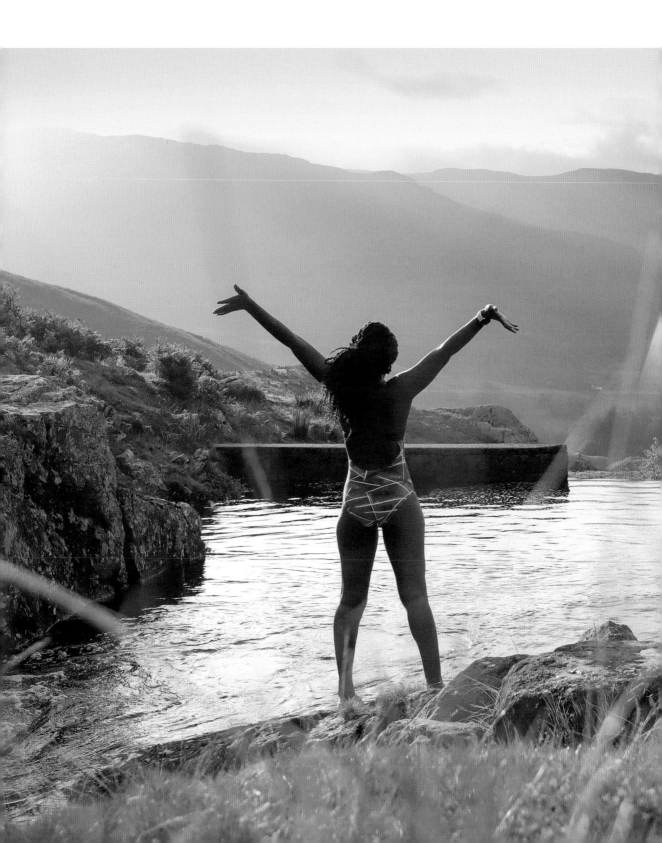

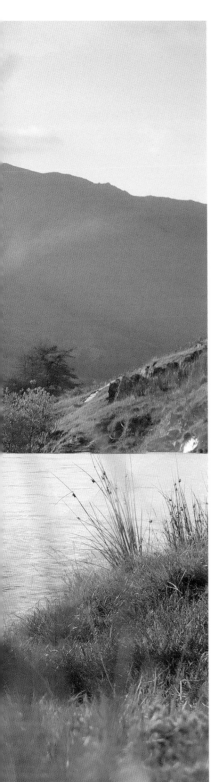

CHAPTER 10

WHERE MIGHT OUTDOOR SWIMMING TAKE YOU?

Now you've started your outdoor swimming journey, have you thought about where it might take you? Adventures and exciting challenges beckon. There are races to sign up to, swimming holidays to escape to, volunteering opportunities where you can give back, and even jobs and careers. Let this chapter inspire you.

MASS PARTICIPATION EVENTS AND RACES

Signing up for an event is a common way to get started in outdoor swimming. Outdoor swimming events have been a big part of my summers for years. With so many on the calendar now, the biggest problem is choosing which ones to do. I like to opt for a mixture of old familiar ones and new ones in places I haven't visited before.

> ### 5 reasons to do a mass participation swimming event
>
> 1. The opportunity to swim somewhere you couldn't normally access.
> 2. The challenge of tackling a long-distance swim with full safety support.
> 3. The excitement of racing and the reward of physically pushing your limits.
> 4. The atmosphere and camaraderie of being part of something challenging.
> 5. The possibility of raising funds for a good cause.

If you're new to outdoor swimming, you might think that events are only for elite, super-fit swimmers. That is almost always not the case. For most swimmers, it's about completion rather than competition. I've been at events where the finishing times for a 1.6km (1-mile) swim ranged from under 20 minutes to as much as two hours. As far as I could tell, swimmers at both ends of the speed spectrum, and everywhere in between, enjoyed their swim.

Everyone is welcome at events and can do the swims in the way they want. However, a small number of events put in time limits. These are usually for safety reasons – for example, a changing tide – so it's worth checking. In those cases where time limits are in place, they are usually generous.

In a normal year, there are hundreds of events around the world. In the UK, most mass participation swims are held between May and September. Popular distances are 1.6km (1 mile), 5km (3.1 miles) and 10km (6.2 miles). The latter is often referred to as the marathon distance of swimming as it's the distance featured in the Olympics and it takes elite swimmers a little under two hours to complete – similar to the time for an elite runner to cover 42.4km (26.2 miles).

You can find event listings for both UK and international swims on the *Outdoor Swimmer* website.

Training for an Event

One reason people do events is to try to swim a distance they haven't done before. Or, if they have done it previously, they might be hoping for a faster time, or maybe to beat their friends. Whatever the reason, you will have a better experience if you do some training first. Training sounds like hard work, but it doesn't have to be. Really, it's just an excuse to do more swimming and it can be a lot of fun. Take a look at Chapter 9 for some suggestions on improving your swim speed and fitness.

MY STORY

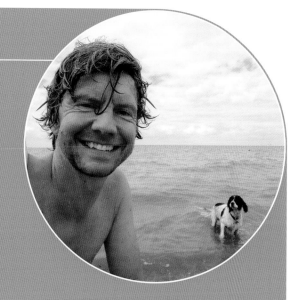

A lifelong love of the water

I have always loved the water. Swimming in the sea on holiday is one of my enduring childhood memories: playing in the waves; exploring coves; jumping off rocks. The same as I love doing now!

In 2009, I did my first organised open water swim – the Great North Swim in Windermere. It was a mile, I loved, it and immediately wanted to do more. At that point it was about events, times and training; other years about challenges; at the moment it is the daily dip. Early morning swims with friends, a wild swim at lunchtime to punctuate the day, or an evening dip as the sun drops down behind the fells. Sunshine, rain, mist, snow – the weather doesn't matter, it's the company and the experience that makes it special.

Although there is nothing I love more than the freedom of summer swimming, for me winter swimming is something truly special. The rush of icy water becomes a craving, whether it is breaking the ice for a short dip or swimming to your limits, pitting your body against the cold. Friendships are made huddled round flasks while dancing around to warm up after a swim – the shared joy of cold water and being outdoors in nature.

It is a joy that I share with others as editor of Outdoor Swimmer magazine, and now as a swim coach I am enjoying introducing even more people to the open water.

JONATHAN COWIE

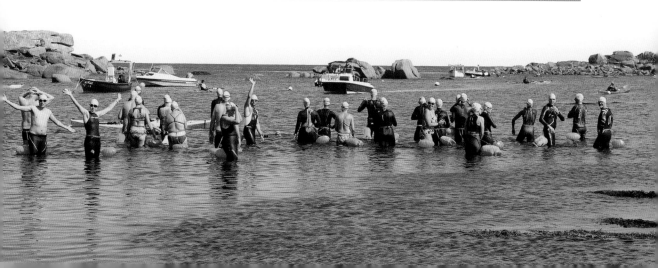

Event Day Preparation

It sounds obvious, but you do need to prepare and plan for events. I've been to lots and it's not uncommon to see people turning up who haven't even unpacked their wetsuit or paid attention to the instructions. I'm sometimes guilty of this myself. I go to so many events that I think I've got everything covered and sometimes I haven't. It's not only embarrassing, but it also results in a worse swim – or even missing the swim completely.

Pre-event check list

1. Put the time and date in your calendar. Organise any accommodation and transport in good time.
2. Think through what you want to get out of the event. Is it a nice day out or a weekend away somewhere new with a swim thrown in? Are you raising funds for charity? Are you looking for nice photos for your social media feeds? Or are you going to race and swim as fast as you can? A little planning can help ensure you achieve what you want.
3. Read event reports and reviews to give you an idea of what to expect. If you won't be able to see the swim course before the event, study it on a map. Is there anything you can look out for that will give you an idea of how far you've swum?
4. Make a plan for how you will swim the event. How much effort will you put into each section? Will you start fast and try to race all the way through, or take it easier to begin with and see how you feel later? If it's a longer swim (say 5km/3.1 miles or more), what and when will you eat during the swim and how will you carry it if nutrition isn't provided by the organiser?
5. Check the car parking arrangements. Some events operate a park and ride or park and walk scheme. Allow enough time for this. If you need a disabled parking space, ask if the organiser can arrange one, and check the distance and terrain you need to cover to get to the start.
6. Make sure you understand the event's wetsuit policy and prepare accordingly.
7. Get your kit ready at least 24 hours in advance and check nothing is broken. Check if any kit is compulsory and make sure you have it or can buy or borrow it at the event.
8. What will you eat on the morning of your swim, in the time leading up to it (if it's not in the morning) and afterwards? Prepare anything you need. Also, decide when you will eat.
9. Check the weather forecast to ensure you have the right clothes for before and after.
10. Find out where and when you need to register and what time you need to be at the briefing, if there is one. Will you need to show photo ID? Are there any disclaimers or online forms to complete in advance?

Events can be stressful experiences. You have to be in the right place at the right time and you will probably push yourself physically. Why add to the stress with poor planning? A little bit of stress can improve your race performance. Too much is detrimental. You will be under enough stress just standing on the start line. Don't ruin the experience by adding unnecessary additional stress.

Event day kit list

I recommend making a kit list for every event. You can use this one as a guide, but it will be better to make your own.

- ☐ Directions to the event
- ☐ Identification
- ☐ Any medication you need to have with you plus MedicAlert if needed
- ☐ Swimming costume, plus spare
- ☐ Goggles, plus spares (maybe have one clear and one tinted pair so you can choose depending on the conditions)
- ☐ Anti-fog spray (or baby shampoo)
- ☐ Swimming cap (it's always good to have your own, even if the event provides one)
- ☐ Petroleum jelly is useful to act as a barrier against chafing on non-wetsuit swims, particularly in sea swims. Put it under your arms and between your thighs. Put some on your chin if it's stubbly as that can rub your arm when you're breathing

- ☐ Wetsuit and wetsuit-safe anti-chafe cream if it's a wetsuit swim
- ☐ Any other accessories you use in the swim (rash vest, neoprene socks, cap, gloves, earplugs, nose clip)
- ☐ Tow float if needed for the swim
- ☐ Any food and drink you need before, during or after your swim
- ☐ Towel
- ☐ Flip-flops or similar
- ☐ Changing robe (optional)
- ☐ Spare warm clothes you can keep on over your costume until the start
- ☐ Warm clothes and coat for after your swim
- ☐ Kit bag
- ☐ Money or cards for post-swim food and celebrations

On the Day

Having read the above, you've arrived at your event in good time and in an excited but confident frame of mind. This means you will already be in a great position for an enjoyable and successful swim. Use the event day check list below to get the most from your day.

Event day check list

1. Complete registration if necessary and collect your swim cap and timing chip if provided. Put your timing chip in a safe place. You could even put it on immediately to ensure you don't misplace it.

2. Check out the start location and the swim route. If the finish is somewhere different to the start, and you have time and access, it's worth checking that, too. As well as route marker buoys, look for any landmarks that could help with navigation.

3. Find some space for doing a gentle warm-up and some mobility exercises. This is especially important if you've had a long journey. You don't need to break sweat, but you should get moving. Arm swings, trunk rotations and leg swings are good.

4. Change into your swimming costume and wetsuit if you're using one. Pull on a warm layer or two over your costume once you've changed so you don't get chilled. You may also need to do this when wearing a wetsuit on a cold day.

5. Once changed, you can continue warming up with some higher-intensity exercises. I like to use stretch cords to mimic the action of swimming (note that mostly you will not be able to do an in-water warm-up). You could continue with the arm swings and add in some star jumps and press-ups.

6. Make sure you attend the swim briefing, if there is one, and re-read the instructions.

7. Review your swim plan and make sure it's still relevant given the conditions on the day.

8. Head to the start in good time. Remind yourself of all the preparation you've done and expect the swim to go well.

9. During the swim, remember your plan and stick to it as well as you can. If your plan is to start steady, don't get caught up in the excitement and sprint off.

10. Remind yourself how lucky you are. You get to swim, hopefully somewhere beautiful or interesting. Relax, stay in the moment, enjoy the surroundings and the weightless feeling of swimming with its unique movement patterns. Pay attention to your effort level and its appropriateness for the distance you are swimming.

11. You can lose a lot of time on a swim if you go off course. Check frequently that you're on the right route.

12. Make sure you finish correctly. You may have to swim under an arch or finish banner, for an in-water finish, or you may have to leave the water and cross a timing mat on land.

13. Stand up carefully after your swim. The effort of swimming combined with being horizontal for a period of time may make you dizzy. Use a handrail if there's one available.

14. Remember to smile for any post-swim pictures.

15. Wash your hands and face before eating or drinking anything.

TYPES OF START

There are several variations on the start theme. Make sure you know how it will work at your event so you can prepare accordingly.

In-water Starts

For an in-water start, you will be asked to enter the water a couple of minutes before the start signal and make your way to the start line, which will usually be in deep water. The organiser will then sound a horn or similar when it's time to start. Sometimes you get a 10-second warning, but not always.

To start fast, get yourself horizontal in the water and scull in place until the start signal. Then, kick hard and do a few fast strokes to build momentum before settling into your usual rhythm. If you're not bothered about starting fast, simply tread water or float until it's time to go. A wetsuit will keep you comfortably afloat.

For non-wetsuit swimmers, an in-water start can be uncomfortable if you have to hang around in the water getting cold. This is most likely to happen at events that have wetsuit and non-wetsuit swimmers, where the wetsuit swimmers are less bothered by the temperature. If you're not wearing a wetsuit, enter the water as close to the start time as possible so you can stay warm for longer.

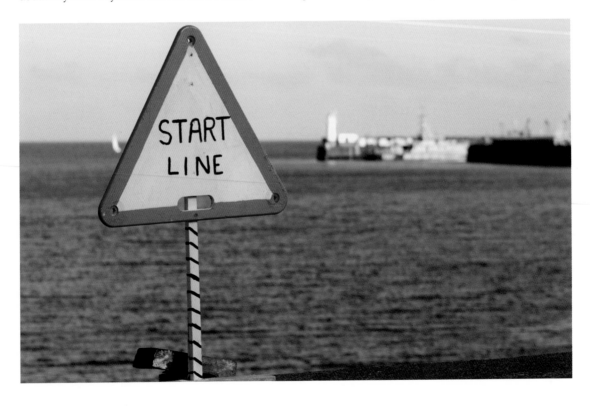

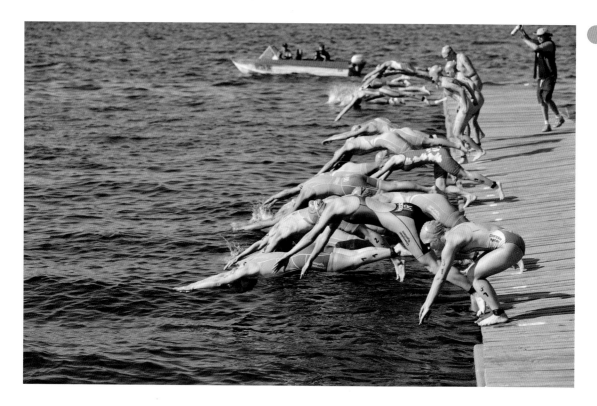

Beach Starts

At beach-start swims, you start on land and run, wade or walk into the water until it's deep enough to swim. I've done beach starts in both sea and lake swims. I can't think of a river swim with a beach start, but it could be done. Sometimes the beach is a temporary man-made carpet-covered ramp in the water.

There are various techniques for those who want to start fast, including swinging your legs outwards while running in for more clearance and, when the water is deep enough, jumping off the bottom into a dive and repeating until it's quicker to swim. Only do these dolphin dives if you know there are no rocks or underwater obstacles. Alternatively, wade in at your own pace and swim when it feels right.

If the event has a beach start, but you need assistance, or you need to start in the water, let the organiser know.

Dive Starts

You mostly find dive starts at elite open water events and some national level championship events, including those for masters swimmers. Competitors line up on a pontoon and dive in as they do in a pool race. If you do ever come across a dive start race and you're not confident about doing a racing dive, you can either jump in (I've seen some elite level swimmers do this) or start in the water.

Mass Starts

Before Covid-19, most outdoor swimming events had what is known as a mass start. A large group of swimmers – sometimes more than 100 – would be bunched into a small space and would all attempt to start swimming at the same time. It's a habit that was adopted from triathlon. For some swimmers, it's a fun and exciting way to start a swim. For others, it's stressful and off-putting.

During the pandemic and its aftermath, some organisers experimented with rolling starts to increase social distancing – one swimmer starting at a time – and these proved popular so may be retained. If you have a preference for one over the other, it's worth checking in advance.

Personally, I think it would be a shame if mass starts disappeared completely as one of things I love about outdoor swimming events is the tactical nature of the racing. A rolling start turns it into a time trial, without the excitement of head-to-head racing. Hopefully, both options will exist in future to keep everyone happy.

Mass starts can be used with both beach and in-water starts. In both cases, you need a plan. Do you want to be in the thick of the action, with a chance of catching a draft (*see* Drafting and pack swimming opposite) from the fast swimmers at the front, or do you want space

and serenity? If it's the former, place yourself on the front row close to the people you want to keep an eye on. Otherwise, hang back.

A mass start is hectic. People, mostly unintentionally, will collide with you, swim over your feet, hit you and possibly dislodge your goggles. I saw one swimmer at the end of a race with his goggles half-filled with blood. Someone had kicked him in the eye at the start. He hadn't realised his goggles had cut him, and was puzzled why his vision was blurry until he got to the end and saw what had happened. He thought it was me who kicked him. If it was, I have no recollection of doing it and certainly didn't do it on purpose.

The way I usually deal with mass starts is to put my head down, try to stay calm and follow someone fast. I do my best to ignore anyone swimming into me or clashing arms. I want to save my energy for swimming. It usually only takes a minute or two for things to settle down and the field to open up so you have space to swim normally. Other times, if I want to avoid the mayhem, I'll find a space at the edge of the pack and start at my own pace.

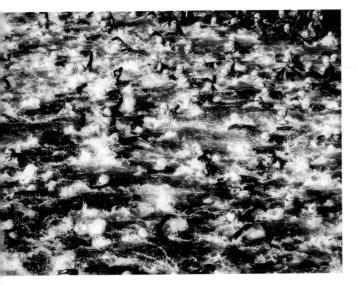

RACE TACTICS

In open water events, there is no compulsion to race. However, if you do want to race, knowing a few tactics can help. You don't need to be at the front of the pack to be racing. These tips will help you to a faster swim wherever you are in the field. They will be useful for triathlon, too, but feel free to skip this section if you have no interest in racing!

Pacing

If you watch an elite swimmer in a long-distance pool race, they will swim every length in almost exactly the same time, except for the first, which is aided by the dive, and maybe the final one or two when they sprint for the finish. It's the same for runners. When Eliud Kipchoge broke the two-hour barrier for a marathon, he ran every kilometre within a few seconds of 2 minutes 50 seconds.

Using an even-pacing strategy for your swim should give the fastest time, but good pacing takes practice. It can feel too easy at the beginning. This tempts you to swim faster, but you will pay for it later and slow down, losing more time than you gained at the beginning.

A good way to practise pacing is to train for it in a pool. When you do a swim with even pacing, the effort feels steady at the start and gradually builds to maximum at the end, while your speed stays the same. An even-pace strategy will usually be your best choice if you're swimming alone or in rolling start events, but there are additional considerations with mass starts.

Drafting and Pack Swimming

Just like geese in formation or cyclists in the Tour de France peloton, swimmers can save energy when swimming in a pack or behind someone else. It may seem counterintuitive that you can save energy by swimming close to someone else as the water is churned up and splashy, but you do.

Drafting is a technique you can use to swim faster (or at the same speed for less effort) by swimming closely behind someone's feet, or to one side with your head roughly level with their hip. If there are more people around you, the effort-saving can be even greater, as long as you don't waste energy in fighting for space.

The easiest way to draft another swimmer is to swim directly behind them. You can get a drafting benefit even if you are 2–3m (6.6–9.9ft) behind, but the energy saving increases the closer you get. Ideally, you want to be far enough behind to not touch their feet, as having someone touching your toes while you swim is annoying and bad manners, plus it interferes with your own swimming.

Often at open water events, and more so in triathlon, swimmers break into packs of varying speeds. For a fast swim, you want to get in a pack that's slightly faster than you can swim on your own. If you try to join one that's too fast, you will waste energy trying to keep up and will suffer later.

Swimmers will often start faster than their sustainable speed and packs may change speed through the swim as different people take the lead. You therefore have to decide if varying your own pace to keep with the pack is a better or worse strategy than swimming on your own at an even pace.

The best way to get used to swimming in close proximity to other swimmers is to do it often. The more events you do, the more experience you get and the better your judgement becomes.

Open water turns

In mass start events, turns are the next most stressful part after the start. If the swim course is a circuit, the turns are marked by buoys. You will be instructed in the briefing which way you have to swim around them.

Turns are always a pinch point as people aim for the shortest route around them. You may see some swimmers doing a fancy roll on to their back as they make a turn. These can help you maintain momentum and allow you to look around and see where your competitors are, but they are not necessary (and note, they don't work if you're using a tow float). It's usually easier to simply swim around. The inside line is obviously the shortest, but not always the quickest as you may get stalled by other swimmers or squeezed against the turn buoy. You may be more comfortable taking a wider line.

Plan ahead for turns and try to position yourself in the pack accordingly. In competitive situations, swimmers use turns to try to gain advantage over each other. The front swimmers can usually get through a turn faster and may try to use it to open up a gap.

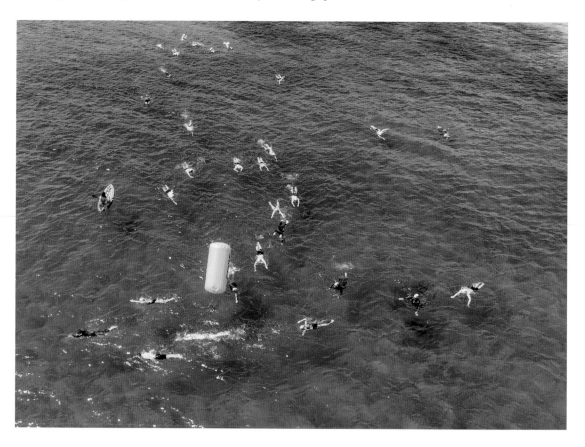

The finish

In elite races, after nearly two hours of swimming, the medal positions are often separated by a few tenths of a second. It all comes down to a sprint finish. Recreational events are usually calmer, but you may find yourself in a sprint finish, even if you're contesting the difference between 50th and 51st. It's surprising how important that can be, especially if you're in a race with a friend or training partner.

As you approach the finish, the pace tends to pick up. Swimmers who have been drafting try to push up alongside the front swimmers. Everyone will be watching each other to see who will jump first to all-out sprint speed. At the same time, they will be jostling for position for the best line to the finish. Start sprinting too soon and you will blow up before the finish. Leave it too late and you will miss your chance. Only experience will teach you the best moment to make your move.

Don't worry that it hurts. It hurts for everyone. When it's time, hit the afterburners and go for it. Don't let up until you cross the finish, whether it's in the water or requires running up the beach. Even if you're falling back, keep pushing. Your competitor might be about to quit and even if they're not, make them work for the win. Some days you'll finish in front and other days not. Either way, you'll have the satisfaction of knowing you did your best.

You may find, approaching the finish, that the field has spread out so much that you're on your own. In which case, there's no need for a sprint finish, unless you want to practise how it feels or to shave a couple of seconds off your time. If you care about these things (and let's face it, we probably shouldn't but often do), it's worth looking around as you approach the finish. It would be annoying to find someone has drafted you for 5km (3.1 miles) and then sprints past you at the end or someone catches you up and overtakes you at the last minute on the side you don't breathe to. It's worth a little effort to stop that happening, isn't it?

As an aside, if you're doing a triathlon, there is no need to sprint at the end. Conserve your energy for the rest of the event.

How to cope when things don't go to plan

Sometimes, your race won't go to plan. The best way to cope is to be prepared. Make a list or think through what could go wrong and how you will deal with it if it does. For example:

- If my goggles fill with water, I will roll on to my back and empty them.
- If I feel panicked, I will swim slowly on my back and focus on breathing until I feel better.
- If I feel like giving up, I will remind myself of how I kept going during that marathon two years ago (choose your own personal example).
- If I get cramp, I will hold on to my tow float and relax until it eases.

LONG-DISTANCE SWIMMING CHALLENGES

Have you ever looked across the water to a speck of land on the horizon and thought, 'I wonder if I could swim there?' If so, maybe marathon swimming is for you.

If you like to think big, then outdoor swimming can offer that, too. The longest mass participation events I know of are the Thames Marathon and the length of Lago d'Orta in Italy, both of which are 14km (8.7 miles) long. There's also the 21km (13-mile) Vidösternsimmet in Sweden, which has fewer participants and is less well known, but is in a beautiful location and worth looking at. These three swims allow wetsuits.

However, most long-distance swimming challenges are swum without a wetsuit as solo efforts, where the swimmer has individual and dedicated boat support. The pinnacle of long-distance swimming is a solo crossing of the English Channel – there are longer, colder and more difficult swims, but the English Channel is the best known and most popular.

There are also shorter, easier and cheaper swims. Some of these, such as the British Long Distance Swimming Association's (BLDSA) length of Windermere are swum in event format with all competitors starting at the same time. However, due to the difficulty and length of the swim, every swimmer is required to have a kayak or rowing boat next to them throughout.

Long-distance marathon swimmers tend to regard wetsuits as unfair assistance and organising bodies either refuse to recognise swims completed in wetsuits, or classify them separately to those done under traditional rules in just a swimming costume, goggles and cap. Part of the challenge is coping with the cold for many hours.

The men's world record for an English Channel crossing is held by Australian Trent Grimsey, who crossed in 6 hours 55 minutes in 2012. The fastest female swimmer is Czech Yvetta Hlaváčová, with a time of 7 hours and 25 minutes. At the other end of the scale, Jackie Cobell took 28 hours and 44 minutes. Most swimmers take between around 12 and 18 hours, with the weather often having a big impact on speed.

If swimming the English Channel is on your bucket list then you will need to do a serious amount of training and preparation, which is beyond the scope of this book, but *see* Further reading and references on pp. 202–203 for other sources of information and advice.

I'd also recommend looking at the events organised by the BLDSA. Swum under traditional Channel swim rules, they offer a range of distances from 1km (0.6 miles) up to 34.8km (21.6 miles) along the length of Loch Lomond (or two laps of Windermere, depending on the year). Many a successful marathon swimmer has built their long-distance swimming experience through BLDSA events. They are also great events in their own right. Look out for the brutal Champion of Champions format, which consists of three swims in one day of 8km (5 miles), 4.8km (3 miles) and 1.6km (1 mile), with a short break in between.

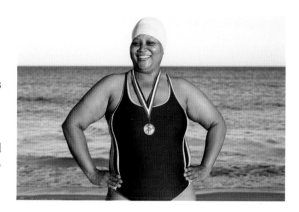

MY STORY

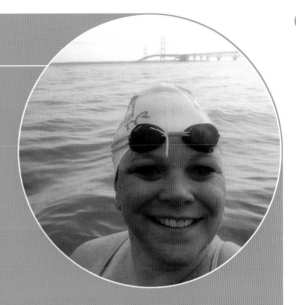

Marathon swimmer

Swimming is my life and any water – no matter how cold, salty or rough it might be – will do.

I got into marathon swimming in 2006 when someone dared me to take on the 12.9km (8-mile) Boston Light Swim. After that, I was completely hooked. By 2009, I'd completed the Triple Crown of Marathon Swimming (the English Channel, the Catalina Channel and the Manhattan Island Marathon Swim) and also become the director of the Boston Light Swim. In 2014, I became the first person to swim the 52km (32.3-mile) length of Lake Pend Oreille and, in 2015, the third American to swim the 35.7km (22.2-mile) length of Loch Ness.

Despite water being my happy place since childhood, growing up in New Jersey, I'd never have guessed back then where the sport would take me. I've seen parts of the world I otherwise would have missed, made friends I otherwise wouldn't have known and been able to create a livelihood as a writer and editor that provides me with purpose.

Still, I do sometimes think back to my summer after graduation when I took a summer lifeguarding position with the Long Beach Township Beach Patrol and, to this day, it's the best job I ever had. I occasionally flirt with the idea of going back one summer, now that I'm in my mid-40s, to see if I can resuscitate the 20-something, Baywatch, babe I used to be...

ELAINE HOWLEY

SWIMMING HOLIDAYS

Swimming holidays have grown in popularity over the past few years and cater for a wide range of abilities and interests.

Going swimming while on holiday has long traditions. Going on holiday to do a series of outdoor swims is a newer concept. But why not? People go on cycling, skiing and hiking holidays. Simon Murie launched SwimTrek in 2003 and created a new swimming holiday industry. SwimTrek now offers swimming holidays to more than 40 destinations and has competition from several other tour operators.

Things to look out for when booking a trip include daily swim distances, likely water temperature and any expectations of swimming ability. Some trips cater for beginners or near beginners while others are hard-core training camps for people preparing for marathon swims. Also check the accommodation options. Will you need to share a room if travelling alone or pay a single supplement, for example? Or if your partner is a non-swimmer, can they join the trip – and if they do, what will they do while you're swimming?

What to Expect from Your Swim Guides

One of the advantages of an organised trip with an experienced operator is the opportunity to swim with guides who have detailed local knowledge. Not only do they know which are the best swims for the weather and tide conditions, but they can also find the friendliest bars and restaurants. They will be able to adapt swims to suit the needs of the group, finding sheltered shallow bays for nervous swimmers or extended routes for faster, more experienced ones.

Swimming in Cornwall and Scilly

I went on a swimming trip to Cornwall and the Isles of Scilly that included travel between swim spots and accommodation on a boat. As my first time aboard a sailing ship, this was a boating as well as a swimming adventure.

Starting in Penzance, we made our way along the southern Cornish coast, swimming two or even three times per day in stunning secluded bays and around dramatic headlands. We then sailed to the Isles of Scilly for more swims between islands, sometimes combined with walks across the islands. With all food provided (and great food too), all we guests had to do was eat, swim, relax and sleep. As someone who loves swimming, eating and sleeping, there isn't much else you could ask for. As a bonus, we saw seals and had a pod of dolphins following the boat and dancing in the bow wave.

The sea around the Isles of Scilly is notoriously cold. I wore a wetsuit for most of my swims. Some others on the trip didn't and had no trouble with the temperature. Luckily, on a swimming holiday you can choose to swim how you feel most comfortable.

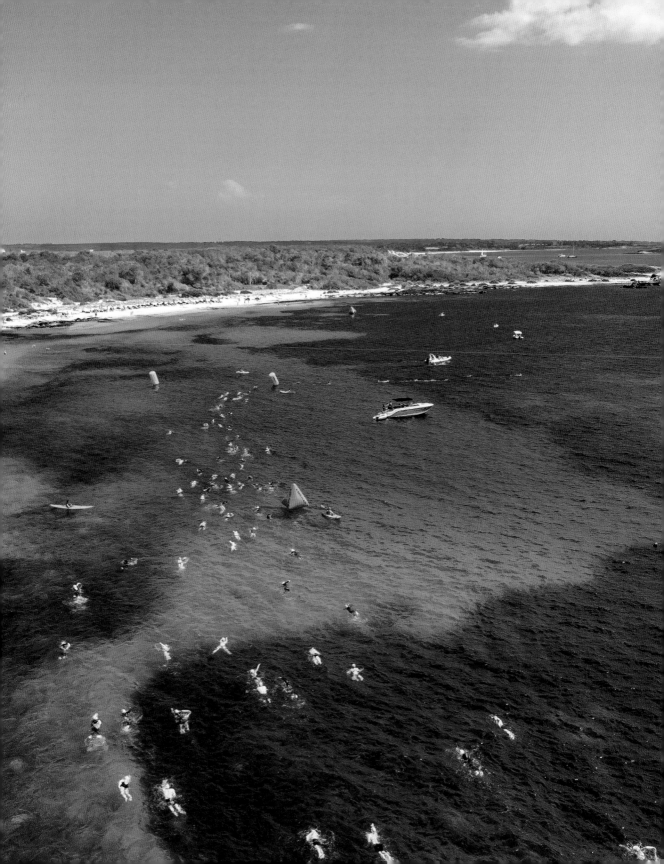

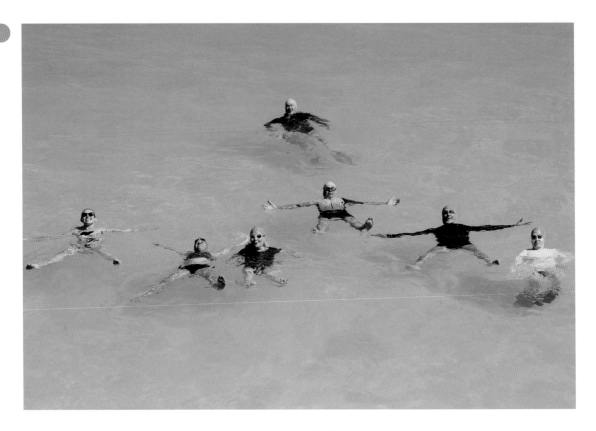

Many guides are strong swimmers themselves, and some are coaches or swim teachers and can therefore advise you on how to improve your swimming. Your swim guides will also be qualified beach lifeguards and will look after your safety in the water. On the trips I've been on, the guides went out of their way to ensure a constant supply of food (very important when you're doing a lot of swimming) and tea and coffee.

Special Kit For Swimming Holidays

It's always best to check with your trip organiser if they have a recommended trip kit list. Depending on the location, this might include waterproof (and reef-safe) sunscreen, long-sleeved swim-vests for sun protection and water shoes for scrambling over rocks. If you're nervous about the water temperature, it's better to have a wetsuit with you just in case, rather than be miserable all week without it.

Do It Yourself Swimming Holidays

One of my favourite things to do is to book a swimming event in another country and build a holiday around it. This works well for a long weekend, but you could easily make a longer holiday out of it. On an organised swimming holiday, all you usually need to do is to get to the right airport. Everything else is sorted. When you go alone, you have to arrange everything yourself. This can be challenging when it comes to event briefings in a language you don't understand, but swims everywhere follow a similar pattern. Just keep an eye on the other swimmers, do what they do and you should be fine.

Swim Festivals

In my experience, the safety provision at events around Europe, and also Turkey and the Middle East, is at a similar level to what you find at a race in the UK, but do pay extra attention to safety briefings and ask for a translation if you're unsure of anything. Also, check your travel and medical insurance. Swimming isn't usually listed as an exclusion, but read the small print, just in case.

If you like open water swimming events and travel, check out BEST Fest in Mallorca. This usually takes place at the end of May and beginning of June and has seven or eight events over the course of a week. You can do as many or as few as you like. In November, look out for the Barbados Open Water Festival, which runs for five days and offers a combination of races and practice swims.

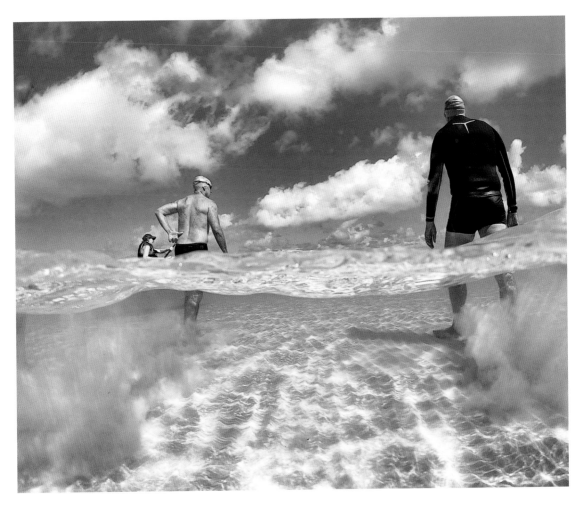

FAMILY SWIMMING

Swimming is an activity that every generation in a family can enjoy together. Taking swimming outside adds to the fun but there are a few additional things you need to take into account to ensure everyone stays safe and enjoys themselves.

Research from Swim England consistently shows that only around half of pupils meet the swimming standards required in the national curriculum – and those standards are basic. Globally, WHO says drowning is the third leading cause of unintentional death. Learning to swim – or at least float and self-rescue – at an early age really could save your life.

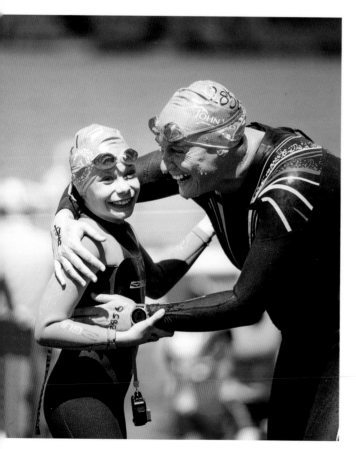

But swimming is so much more than a life-saving skill. Being water confident opens up a lifetime of opportunities for fun and adventure, both through swimming and other watersports. However, swimming lessons are expensive, and swimming often isn't taught in schools, or limited resources mean it is taught badly.

So what can parents and carers do?

If you can, take your children swimming often. I know this can be tricky because of the cost and pool restrictions on the number of children you can take at a time so you may have to do shifts. If you can, invite the grandparents, too. An extra pair of hands and eyes improves safety. Also, some older family members may find swimming easier to join in with than, say, a kick-around in the park. Get everyone in the water and have fun. Make it play time for everyone. Do underwater handstands, dive for objects on the bottom, play tag. As your children get older, allow them to invite friends along. Get lessons, if your children want them and you can afford them, but I think having water fun together will give them a better start.

When it comes to swimming outdoors, it's more likely kids will want to play and have fun rather than swim – swimming is just a skill to make everything else possible. Find sheltered beaches (both inland and at the sea) or rock pools where they experience natural water safely. Let them enjoy the sensation of cool, natural water on their skin and being knocked about by waves. Older family members can also join the fun outdoors. My mum used to enjoy bodyboarding with my children when they were younger.

MY STORY

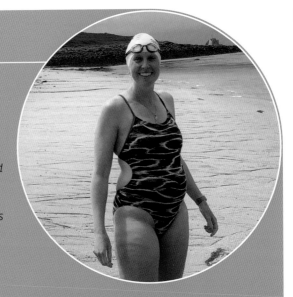

Swimming while pregnant

I swam right up until my due date in a swimming pool, although by the end I was considerably slower than when I started! I swam outdoors too but tended to limit it to short dips or until I felt the babies kicking hard (you read that right, I said 'babies' as I had twins). One time I was on a trip to the Scilly Isles and the water was around 13 degrees. I think they must have felt the cold as they started kicking after only a couple of minutes. Throughout my pregnancy, I was careful about where I swam and avoided places where I had doubts about the water quality.

When it comes to swimming during pregnancy, I heard a lot of varied advice. In the end, I think it comes down to what you're comfortable doing. Certainly, by the end of my pregnancy, getting into the water was the only place I felt any kind of relief and weightlessness as I'd put on around 20kg (3.5 stone).

The other thing to consider is getting back into swimming after childbirth. I naively thought I'd be able to get straight back to where I was before until I realised it takes a long time to recover. My abs were completely shot, for example, so swimming felt really strange to start with.

ALICE TODD

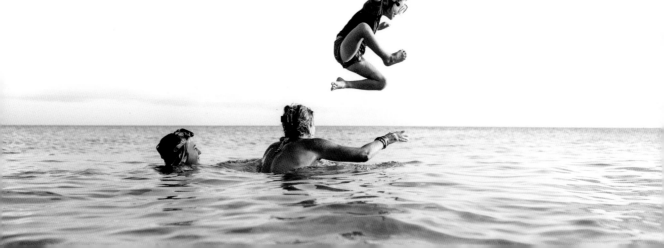

Safety

Children get colder quicker than adults and, if they are having fun, they might not notice. Be ready with warm towels and plenty of layers, and intervene sooner rather than later if you think they are getting cold (for example, if their lips turn blue or they start shivering). Also, make sure they are protected from the sun. The usual parenting stuff.

Test anywhere your children are swimming first. Make sure there are no sudden changes in depth that might catch them unawares. While waves are fun, children are more easily knocked off their feet than adults and may be dragged towards deeper water. Stay close at all times. For small children or weak swimmers, ideally, you should have a ratio of one adult for every child. And of course, look out for rip tides and currents, and adhere to all the normal safety considerations for swimming outdoors.

Because outdoor swimming is something that people of all ages can do, it's a great equaliser and an activity that families with children of different ages can often enjoy together. Some of the best family holidays I've had involved getting a wild swimming guidebook for a region and finding places to swim.

Family Events

If you enjoy swimming events, it's possible your children might want to give them a go too. You will need to look around for family-friendly events. This is harder than it sounds as many events have cut-offs at ages 18 or 16. However, there are a few that allow children as young as eight. These sometimes require a parent or carer to swim alongside the youngest children. Two that I know of are Henley Swim and Great Swim. These family-friendly events offer children an outdoor swimming experience rather than a race, which makes them suitable and accessible for both recreational and club swimmers.

If your child is a competitive club swimmer and wants to race then look for open water events sanctioned by your local national governing body. These events are usually only open to club swimmers and the standard is often high. As most pool events are sprints, or middle distance at best, open water gives an opportunity for those who are better at endurance to shine. The excitement of an outdoor swimming experience can also keep older children interested in club swimming. Since marathon swimming became an Olympic event in 2008, clubs have shown more interest in open water swimming.

Top tip:

Look out for programmes such as Swim Safe. This is a free outdoor swimming and water safety programme for children aged 7–14 created by Swim England and the Royal National Lifeboat Institution. Courses are held through the summer at around 40 beaches and inland water locations. Each session lasts about an hour, introduces children to open water safety and gives them an in-water experience.

GIVING BACK TO THE OUTDOOR SWIMMING COMMUNITY

It's always good to share and if it's a pastime you're evangelical about, like outdoor swimming, it's even better.

Involve Others

Once you discover outdoor swimming and the beneficial impact it has on your life, it's natural to want to share it, and introduce more people. At its simplest level, this might involve inviting a friend to your next swim and providing reassurance while they experience cold water shock for the first time or sharing their delight when they realise the cold isn't the barrier they thought it would be.

You may find, after you've introduced a few people, that you have started a little group, possibly by accident. You might then ask yourself if you should widen 'membership' to people you don't yet know, perhaps by starting a Facebook group.

Some caution is needed. Make it clear that any swims you organise are done so in a voluntary capacity, and that any swimmer taking part should make their own risk assessment and must take sole responsibility for the risks they are taking while swimming. Incidentally, the same applies to you if you join a swim organised by another group – always do your own risk assessment and take responsibility for your own safety.

Before creating a group, check Facebook, the Bluetits' website and the Outdoor Swimming Society's wild swim groups listings. If there is already a group in your area doing the swims you want to do, there's no need to create a new one. And once you have some outdoor swimming experience, if there is already a local group, I'm sure they would welcome any extra voluntary support.

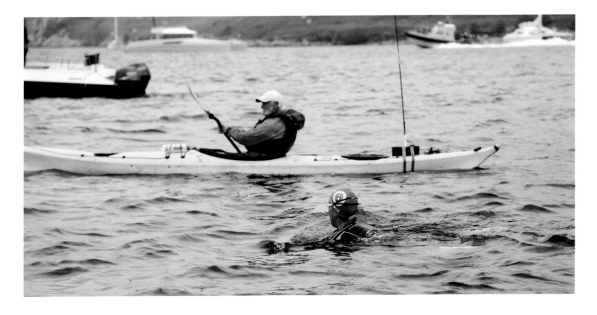

Event volunteers

Swimming events always need help with registration, marshalling people to the right place and clearing up afterwards. Volunteers aren't usually paid, but sometimes receive a free lunch, a T-shirt or free entry into a future event, plus the feel-good factor of helping out and facilitating the enjoyment of other swimmers. Volunteering is a great way to stay involved and experience the buzz of an event if you can't swim for some reason, such as an injury. And sometimes it's just more fun standing on the sidelines watching other people swim than getting in the water yourself. If you're interested in volunteering, check out the event organiser's website for details on how to apply. Alternatively, send the organiser an email.

If you are an experienced kayaker or SUPer, you may also be asked to provide on-water support at an event. Or you can volunteer to escort your friends for a swim. Some days, I'd rather be on the river than in it, so I'll bring out a SUP and paddle alongside my friends as they swim. I find it soothing, listening to the rhythm of their swimming. You can also take great photos and videos from a SUP, which your swimmers will appreciate. In addition, you are a more visible presence on the water in a kayak or on a SUP than in the water and you can see further. This helps you keep the swimmers safe. You can also carry snacks and other kit for them.

Open Water or Beach Lifeguard Qualifications

Events and venues frequently need lifeguards as well as volunteers. Becoming a lifeguard will give you more volunteering opportunities as well as the possibility of paid work if that's something you're looking for. The two main qualifications in the UK are the RLSS Open Water Lifeguard and National Vocational Beach Lifeguard Qualification. The first is for lifeguards who provide cover in non-tidal water and is ideal for those lifeguarding at supervised inland venues or swimming events in lakes. The beach lifeguard qualification is the one you need if you want to work as a lifeguard on UK beaches. If you ever want to work as a guide on a swimming holiday, a beach lifeguard qualification is usually required.

Other countries will have their own associations providing lifeguard training. For example, check out the Australian Lifeguard Service and the American Lifeguard Association.

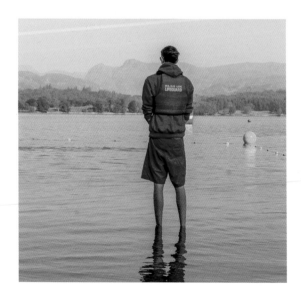

MY STORY

City Boy turned swimming guide

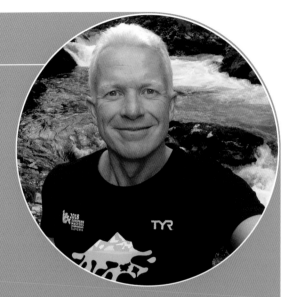

After 30-plus years of corporate life an opportunity came my way to give up my suits, emails, meetings, deadlines and daily commutes. Corporate life had treated me well and enabled me to work with many wonderful people, but I had grown tired of it and needed a complete change. I had no real plan, just a personal mission statement: 'To work in, on and around water.' I gave myself a year to make the transition.

Growing up, I had been a competitive swimmer and at the height of my swim career represented England and Great Britain in open water, so I had a lot of swimming experience, but no relevant qualifications. My first task was to take some courses, including ones in: swim teaching, swim coaching, open water coaching, lifeguarding (pool, open water and beach), powerboat, VHF radio and first aid.

I love being able to teach people to swim, the joy when they believe they can do it, their first float, first strokes, first jump, the fun and the laughter. I also help to keep people safe at events; watching people achieve their own personal challenges for whatever reason is great to see. I didn't know where I would end up when I started this journey, but I found my dream job working for a swimming holiday company as a guide. They send me to locations around the world, usually remote places, planning swims and providing safety cover for groups of swimmers with the help of local pilots. I have learnt so much and am still learning about the weather, the sea, marine life and so much more. I am living the dream and having lots of fun and laughter with likeminded people from all corners of the world.

SIMON EMM

Coaching

Taking things a step further, how about training to become an open water swimming coach? Coaching in outdoor swimming encompasses everything from helping people overcome their fears and doing their first tentative strokes to preparing for races or major swimming challenges. Some coaches work as volunteers with their local clubs or groups, while others go on to set up coaching businesses.

Depending on what pre-qualifications and swimming experience you have, a coaching course can be done over a period of a couple of weekends and involves a mixture of classroom learning and practical in-water sessions. Where you take it from there depends on you.

In the UK, there are two main routes to becoming an open water coach, either through the Institute of Swimming (IoS) or the Swimming Teachers' Association (STA). The IoS option (Level 2 Coaching Open Water Swimming) is an add-on qualification for people who are already swimming coaches or teachers. The STA option (Open Water Swimming Coaching) has similar course prerequisites, but also offers an alternative entry route for people who are not previously qualified swimming coaches or teachers. In this case, you need to demonstrate your open water experience and knowledge through an online upskill programme.

Campaigning

Two of the most frequent questions outdoor swimmers ask are: (1) is it clean; and (2) is it legal? As discussed elsewhere in this book, sadly our waterways are sometimes polluted, and swimmers' rights of access are limited and unclear. As more people add their voices to various campaigns on both of these issues, greater pressure is put on water companies, landowners and politicians to reduce pollution and improve access.

Groups to look out for and support include:

SWIM ENGLAND
Campaigning for better access and increased safety for open water swimmers (www.swimming.org/openwater/outdoor-pledge)
BRITISH CANOEING
Clear Access, Clear Waters campaign (https://clearaccessclearwaters.org.uk)
SURFERS AGAINST SEWAGE
Various campaigns (www.sas.org.uk)
THE LONDON WATER KEEPER
Campaigning for a Thames fit to swim in (www.londonwaterkeeper.org.uk)

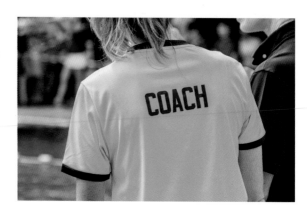

Also look out for local groups who might be campaigning on various issues. For example, swimmers successfully campaigned to have the River Wharfe in Ilkley, Yorkshire, designated as a Bathing Water, which imposed additional testing and water quality requirements on the Environment Agency and Yorkshire Water. This was the first time a local group had successfully campaigned for Bathing Water Status for a river in England and therefore marked a major milestone in citizen action for cleaner rivers.

Take part in beach cleans or become a local hero by collecting litter around your nearest swim spot. It doesn't have to be a chore. I spoke to a women I saw collecting litter recently and told her how much I appreciated her efforts. She said there was no need to thank her. She'd started doing it for her mental health and as a reason to get outside every day, and it gave her opportunities to connect and chat with other people.

A few people use outdoor swimming as a campaigning tool. Lewis Pugh is probably the most famous for his swims at extreme latitudes and altitudes, places where the water is supposed to be frozen, but isn't due to climate change. Laura Owen Sanderson set up We Swim Wild as a not-for-profit company and campaigning body to protect wild spaces and wild waters across the UK. She encourages swimmers to combine their hobby with adventure activism to highlight issues in the environment and citizen science. She leads by example through swims in Britain's national parks, where she collects water samples to test for microplastics and other silent contaminates.

Careers in outdoor swimming

As outdoor swimming has become more popular, it has created opportunities for paid employment, whether occasional casual work or full-time employment. These include lifeguarding or managing venues, being a guide on a swimming holiday, working for a swimming holiday company or other business in the sector in, for example, a commercial or marketing position. A number of entrepreneurs have built successful and interesting businesses offering swimming holidays and trips, coaching services and useful kit.

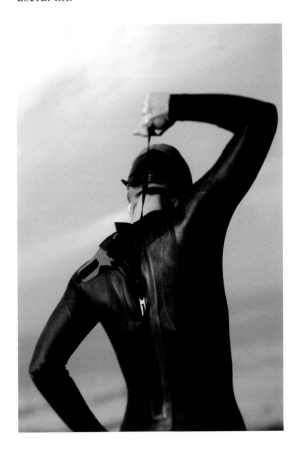

Further reading and references

Classic books

- *Haunts of the Black Masseur: The Swimmer as Hero*, Charles Sprawson, 1992, Vintage UK.
- *Waterlog: A Swimmer's Journey through Britain*, Roger Deakin, 2000, Vintage UK.

Guide books

- *Wild Swim (River, Lake, Lido and Sea: The Best Places to Swim Outdoors in Britain)*, Kate Rew, 2009, Guardian Books.
- *Wild Swimming: 300 Hidden Dips in the Rivers, Lakes and Waterfalls of Britain*, Daniel Start, 2013, Wild Things Publishing. (In addition, Wild Things Publishing has an international series of wild swim guidebooks).
- *Swimming London: 50 Best Pools, Lidos, Lakes and Rivers from Around the Capital*, Jenny Landreth, 2014, Aurum Press.
- *The Lido Guide*, Emma Pusill and Janet Wilkinson, 2019, Unbound.
- *A Guide to Wild Swimming in Cornwall*, Bethany Allen, Max Campbell and Lydia Paleschi, 2021, Kelp Studios LLP.
- *Swimming Wild in the Lake District: The most beautiful wild swimming spots in the larger lakes*, Suzanna Cruickshank, 2020, Vertebrate Publishing.

Swimming technique and training

- *Swim Smooth: The Complete Coaching System for Swimmers and Triathletes*, Paul Newsome and Adam Young, 2012, John Wiley & Sons.
- *Open Water Swimming Manual: An Experts Survival Guide for Triathletes and Open Water Swimmers*, Lynne Cox, 2013, Vintage Books.

- *Open Water: The History and Technique of Swimming*, Mikael Rosén, 2019, Chronicle Books.
- *Total Immersion: The Revolutionary Way to Swim Better, Faster, and Easier*, Terry Laughlin, 1996, Simon & Schuster.

History and general

- *The Story of Swimming*, Susie Parr, 2011, Dewi Lewis Media.
- *Open Water: The History and Technique of Swimming*, Mikael Rosén, 2019, Chronicle Books.
- *Taking the Waters: A Swim Around Hampstead Heath*, Caitlin Davies, 2012, Frances Lincoln Limited.
- *Downstream: A History and Celebration of Swimming the River Thames*, Caitlin Davies, 2015, Autumn Press Ltd.
- *Splash!: 10,000 Years of Swimming*, 2020, Howard Means, Allen & Unwin.

Memoir and miscellaneous

- *Leap In: A Woman, Some Waves and the Will to Swim*, Alexandra Heminsley, 2017, Penguin.
- *I Found My Tribe*, Ruth Fitzmaurice, Vintage (Chatto & Windus).
- *A Boy in the Water*, Tom Gregory, 2018, Particular Books (Penguin).
- *Swimming Against the Stream*, Jean Perraton, 2005, Jon Carpenter Publishing.
- *Taking the Plunge: The Healing Power of Wild Swimming for Mind, Body and Soul*, Anna Deacon and Vicky Allan, 2019, Black & White Publishing.

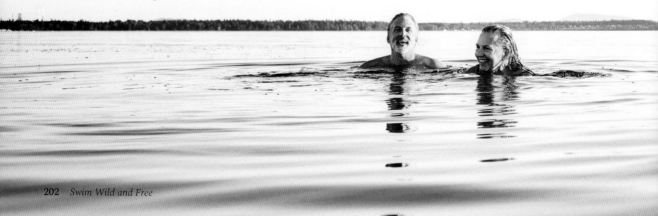

Online resources

- Outdoor Swimmer – www.outdoorswimmer.com
- Venue listings – www.outdoorswimmer.com/venues
- (As well as the listings on the Outdoor Swimmer website, you can also find them through Swim England. The Royal Life Saving Association, British Triathlon and Swim England run a voluntary venue accreditation scheme called Beyond Swim (previously SH_2OUT), which provides additional reassurance to swimmers.)
- Event listings – www.outdoorswimmer.com/events
- UK Beaches – www.thebeachguide.co.uk
- Lifeguarded Beaches (UK) – www.rnli.org/find-my-nearest/lifeguarded-beaches
- The Outdoor Swimming Society – www.outdoorswimmingsociety.com
- Mental Health Swims – www.mentalhealthswims.co.uk
- Swim England – www.swimming.org/swimengland
- Swimming Teachers' Association – www.sta.co.uk
- International Winter Swimming Association – www.iwsa.world
- International Ice Swimming Association – www.internationaliceswimming.com
- Advice for swimmers with disabilities – https://sophie-adaptive-athlete.com (includes map of accessible swimming spots)
- Guide to world sea temperatures – www.seatemperature.org
- The Bluetits (outdoor swimming groups) – thebluetits.co

Swim holiday companies and guides

- SwimTrek – www.swimtrek.com
- SwimQuest – www.swimquest.uk.com
- Strel Swimming Adventures – www.strel-swimming.com
- The Big Blue - https://thebigblueswim.com/
- Swim Vacation – www.swimvacation.com
- Dip Advisor – www.thedipadvisor.co.uk
- Suzanna Swims – www.suzannaswims.co.uk

Scientific and other references

- Benefits of cold water immersion – www.physoc.onlinelibrary.wiley.com/doi/full/10.1113/EP086283
- Outdoor swimming and mental health – https://casereports.bmj.com/content/2018/bcr-2018-225007
- Cold water immersion and Alzheimer's – www.hra.nhs.uk/planning-and-improving-research/application-summaries/research-summaries/the-cold-shock-response-induced-by-cold-water-swimming/
- Static and dynamic immersion in cold water – https://bjsm.bmj.com/content/45/2/e1.2
- 'Autonomic conflict': a different way to die during cold water immersion? – https://physoc.onlinelibrary.wiley.com/doi/full/10.1113/jphysiol.2012.229864
- Swimming-induced pulmonary oedema – www.ncbi.nlm.nih.gov/pmc/articles/PMC6067793/
- Advice on preventing the spread of invasive species – www.nonnativespecies.org/checkcleandry
- Access rights on the River Wye – www.gov.uk/guidance/information-to-help-boaters-on-the-river-wye
- Trends in outdoor swimming – www.outdoorswimmer.com/trends-in-outdoor-swimming

A FEW FINAL THOUGHTS

I barely remember learning to swim. I was about four years old. I went through swimming lessons, joined a swimming club, swam for my town, county and university, and have continued swimming, with only occasional breaks, ever since. I've been on courses, taken one-to-one lessons, read lots of books and blogs and watched countless videos on swimming, and yet I'm still learning. I don't expect I will ever stop.

With all the magazine articles and blog posts I've written about swimming over the years, I know I've written enough words to fill several books. I was therefore delighted Bloomsbury offered me the opportunity to write this one. I did wonder, initially, if I could pull it together from things I'd written previously, but quickly realised it would become disjointed and unwieldy. I therefore started from zero and I'm glad I did as it gave me the chance to talk to all the wonderful people whose stories appear in these pages. I hope those gave you a flavour of the many different directions swimming can take you.

This book, like any other, has a page limit and I've had to leave some things out. For example, while we've tried to cover everything you need to start exploring the world of outdoor swimming, unlike many sports books, we've decided not to include detailed training plans. There are a couple of reasons for this. First, in my experience, only a minority of outdoor swimmers want them when they are starting out. Acclimatisation to outdoor water temperatures and overcoming nerves are higher priorities than swimming faster. Second, you can find many training sessions online, free of charge. In addition, I have included some suggestions for designing your own training sessions and plans. If you are setting yourself race and performance goals, creating your own sessions and plans can be really powerful. Also, for similar reasons, I haven't gone into detail about swimming

technique. There are fantastic books already out there that cover swimming technique in great depth. Please *see* Further reading and references on pp. 202–203 for some suggestions on this.

I truly hope that this book has ignited a deep and long-lasting passion for outdoor swimming, and provides you with the information and confidence to fully immerse yourself in this wonderful, life-enhancing activity. There will always be more to learn and explore. If you haven't done so already, I'd encourage you to subscribe to *Outdoor Swimmer* magazine, sign up for its email newsletter and follow it on social media. You can also follow me directly on Twitter @SimonDGriffiths

As a result of writing this book, I asked my mother why she was so keen for me and my siblings to learn to swim as children. She'd never been a competitive swimmer, but says she had enjoyed swimming as a child and had fond memories of school swimming lessons. She grew up in Topsham and remembers, when she was around 11 or 12 years old, taking the train to Exmouth with a friend during summer holidays and spending days splashing around in the sea (there was no helicopter parenting back then). She's now in her 80s and still swims, mostly in the pool in her apartment block in Spain where she lives, but also in the sea when she has somebody else to go with her. One of my ambitions is to keep swimming into my 80s.

ACKNOWLEDGEMENTS

Writing a book, like doing a swim, is far from a solo endeavour. There's always a team in the background, and when thanking them, there's always a danger you forget someone. So many people have helped me on my swimming journey throughout my life I could never list them all, from swimming teachers and coaches to friends and competitors, and later to all the people who helped establish *Outdoor Swimmer*.

First, of course, I want to thank my parents who put me in the water from a young age, spent hours on the poolside while I was training and drove me to competitions and training camps. I know not everyone has that opportunity. My partner and children deserve a big mention, too, for all the swimming trips I've inflicted on them, and for supplying me with essential coffee and chocolate while I've been writing.

Thanks, too, to the amazing team at *Outdoor Swimmer* (Jonathan Cowie, Ella Foote, Luke Chamberlain, Stuart Churchill, Yvonne Turner, Gary Hall and Kirstyn Luton). Without them running the show, I wouldn't have had time to write this book, plus they provided technical help, advice and contacts.

Next on my list are my friends, swimming buddies and coaches at Teddington Swimming Club Masters (TSCM). It really is a brilliant club, in no small part due to a small number of volunteers who run it and skilfully guided it through the Covid-19 pandemic. Overlapping with TSCM but including additional swimmers are the members of various WhatsApp groups I belong to that are dedicated to swimming year round in the Thames. Not only do these people share my swimming adventures, but they also inspire me with their swimming challenges and other athletic endeavours, and several have assisted directly with this book.

Finally, a big thank you to the team at Bloomsbury Sport who guided me through the process of creating my first book. You might have thought publishing a magazine would have given me all the experience I needed to publish a book. Far from it. A book is a different beast and their experience, expertise and enthusiasm has been fantastic.

About the author

Simon Griffiths is the founder and publisher of *Outdoor Swimmer* magazine, which has been running since 2011. He has previously written for *Triathlete's World*, has appeared in the *Telegraph* online, and frequently provides articles and training advice for event organisers and other swimming-related businesses. He was part of the working group that created the STA's Open Water Swimming Coaching qualification. Simon lives in Richmond, Surrey, where he swims outdoors year round and is a member of Teddington Swimming Club Masters.

INDEX